SCAMDEMIC-PLANDEMIC

SCAMDEMIC-PLANDEMIC

Hugh Cameron

Library of Congress Control Number:		2023907357
ISBN:	Hardcover	978-1-6698-7444-7
	Softcover	978-1-6698-7443-0
	eBook	978-1-6698-7442-3

Print information available on the last page.

Rev. date: 04/18/2023

To order additional copies of this book, contact:
Xlibris
844-714-8691
www.Xlibris.com
Orders@Xlibris.com
850948

Contents

Acknowledgments

In this book there are extensive quotations from William Shakespeare, Christopher "Kit" Marlowe, Rudyard Kipling, Virgil, Cicero, Tacitus, Boethius, Edward Fitzgerald, Samuel Coleridge, Lord Tennyson, T. S. Elliot, Francis Thomson, Robert Burns, Rupert Brooke, Ernest Dowson, Oscar Wilde, Sir Henry Newbolt, Dietrich Bonhoeffer, Martin Niemöller, Hegel, Confucius, The King James Version of the Bible, and many others.

Abstract

This is the third book in this series. It is a collection of sequential posts starting in January 2022, almost completely unedited. I have added some comments from readers, often penetrating and acerbic.

In May 2020, we realized, based on the data from the *Diamond Princess* cruise ship that this virus was tightly targeted largely at the ill elderly and that healthy people under age sixty were at almost no risk. We knew that children did not get sick and did not transmit. In fact, without the PCR test, we would not have known there was anything of significance on the loose. This made the subsequent events of 2020 and 2021 inexplicable.

It was inconceivable that the same unnecessary protocols were followed in 2022. The peculiar reaction to the monkeypox was even more inexplicable and the subsequent drumbeat of global warming suggested an ulterior motive. These posts follow the changes in beliefs which may be of historical significance and help avoid a subsequent disaster.

Introduction

The *Rubáiyát* says it all:

> Whether at Naishapur or Babylon,
> Whether the cup with sweet or bitter run,
> The wine of life keeps oozing drop by drop,
> The leaves of life keep falling one by one.
>
> —Omar Khayyám

The relatively harmless coronavirus from Wuhan seems to have been the catalyst to destabilize the West and, perhaps, the rest of the world. Whether the destabilization was by accident or design is as yet unclear. Perhaps it is simply in the nature of civilizations that they all contain telomeres, the seeds of their own destruction. The Enlightenment was wondrous while it lasted, but it is fading into the sunset. As Dowson wrote,

> They are not long, the days of wine and roses.
> Out of a misty dream
> Our path emerges for a while, then closes
> Within a dream.
>
> —"Vitae Summa Brevis Spem Nos Vetat Incohare Longam"

This is the third book in this series dealing with this entirely manmade tragedy. Diseases are part of human existence. They come and go. Typhus, TB, and malaria are still with us, killing millions. Even cholera, an eminently preventable disease, is still present in some countries. It was introduced into Haiti by the UN peacekeepers and continues to devastate that poor, benighted island.

Disease has changed history. There is speculation that it was the introduction of malaria to Italy from Africa, which led to the final collapse of the Western Roman Empire. The Black Death, or bubonic plague, killed almost one-third of Europe and in part, spurred the industrial revolution as the shortage of workers forced an increase in wages, which in turn led to industrialization to replace the missing workers.

Most diseases are well understood, but some, like the Spanish flu, remain shrouded in mystery. No one quite knows where it came from. There have been many theories, some of which once sounded ludicrous, like the one which suggested it was the result of the vaccination of the US troops on the way to Europe with a new vaccine. No one took that particular explanation seriously until the disaster of the last two years, which has shown just how badly things can go wrong.

We do know of the disaster of polio vaccines in various parts of the world. Recently, there have been rumors about the relationship between microcephaly and a new vaccine. The outbreak of microcephaly in Brazil was blamed on the Zika virus. Rumor has it that Zika is endemic to Brazil and has never produced microcephaly in the past, and some cases of microcephaly never had Zika. Furthermore, microcephaly seems to have disappeared.

You see the problem. Given the misinformation provided by governments and the egregious misstatements by the three-letter agencies supposed to protect the people and given the inexplicable banning of repurposed drugs, which, while they might not have been a panacea, were certainly innocuous, who believes what anymore? It is certainly clear that the legacy media is simply a source of propaganda, and their "news" and views are not to be taken seriously.

It has reached the stage where the German Iron Chancellor, Bismarck's statement seems real, that "Something should only be believed when it has been officially denied."

When the Wuhan virus escaped or was released, likely in May 2019, it slowly spread around the world. We know from sewage studies, it was in Europe and Brazil by November 2019. It was almost certainly deliberately spread at the military games in Wuhan in October 2019. In October 2019, a meeting was held in New York, called Event 201. This so clearly predicted exactly what was going to happen that it seems obvious someone knew something.

Nothing much happened until the virus triggered seasonally as many viruses do, early in 2020. Even so, had there been no PCR test, it seems unlikely that anyone would have noticed, as it was no worse than a bad flu year. The results from Africa clearly demonstrate that with no tests and no needles, there was no epidemic. It was not the virus that caused the problem, it was the inexplicable reaction to it, almost as if it had been rehearsed at Event 201. Two years ago, such a statement would have seemed lunacy. But given the unfolding events, who knows?

This book, like the first two, *Journal of the Plague Year* (2020) and *Plague or Pseudo Plague* (2021), consists of sequential posts laying out the history as it unfolded. Given the attempts already to rewrite history, such a chronicle is necessary to document what actually seemed to happen. The reader must continue to bear in mind that censorship was extreme and the writer had to be very circumspect as these posts were clearly frequently shadow-banned, and there were constant fears of deplatforming.

The other fear was that doctors in Canada were warned by their licensing bodies and ministers of health that any disparaging remarks about the government-approved rules, and especially the so-called vaccine, could result in the loss of a medical license. The medical licensing body in Ontario went as far as to suggest to doctors that any patient who refused the vaccine be treated as if they had a mental illness.

In the first two books, I was not allowed to use the words "hydroxychloroquine" and "Ivermectin," as these potentially useful drugs were censored by big tech, so they were referred to as "the drugs which cannot be named." By calling the vaccine the needle, I hoped to avoid the censors. In general, I avoided full names for the same reason, preferring to use the first name only. Most people will know who was being referred to. Free speech is relative. It is not protected at all in Canada and clearly is under assault in the US.

Anyway! On to the tale of the ongoing greatest manmade or Public health disaster in history.

January 3, 2022

A new year! What is the path ahead? Is it "down to Gehenna or up to the throne," or as Mithras said,

"Many roads hast thou fashioned,
all of them lead to the light"?

Miguel de Cervantes of Don Quixote wrote in 1610, "There are two families in this world; the Haves and the Have-nots." The response to this pseudo plague has made that clear, the Zoom class and the rest. Government schools in Ontario are again closed. Private schools are mostly open. Tough on the poor kids. Good for me as the roads are empty when I drive to the clinics.

The pampered Zoom class do not know history. During a civilization collapse, as that seems to be what is happening, they never survive.

Welcome to the world of George Orwell. From *Animal Farm*: "Four legs good, two legs bad" translates to "needled good, un-needled bad." But you gotta run to keep up with them needles. In Israel, it is four needles good, two needles bad. Also, "all animals are equal, but some are more equal than others." In Europe, no needle passport, no work, or shopping for you. The fact that the needle seems to reduce resistance to Omicron (i.e., make infection more likely) is ignored.

In *1984*, Orwell described "Big Brother is watching you." He certainly is via your needle passport. And doublethink; the failed policies of masking and lockdown will be reintroduced, and this time, they will do something.

And think of Oppenheimer, looking at the atomic bomb blast: "[Scientists] have known sin; and this is knowledge which they cannot lose." Despite the number of crazy fingers on the trigger, only two bombs have been dropped in anger on Hiroshima and Nagasaki. The scientific sin was not the bomb, it was Climategate, which revealed to the world that science was being perverted. That was an inflection point as the perversion was ignored, and leaders carried on with the destruction of Western civilization.

This made it fairly easy to use a tightly targeted virus to close down the world. Most people now know that in most countries, year on year, there have been no excess deaths. And yet the charade continues.

There are a few bright lights like Scandinavia and Florida. Will they be enough to withstand the onrushing tide of collectivism? What do you think?

Comments

1. My thoughts you ask. The stupid gets stupider! The gullible get more gullible! The children are punished further; and the elderly, whose time on earth is short, get no visitors, no love, and no last chance to impart wisdom. I cannot thank you enough for being the voice of reason for the last two years. Without it, I thought I was going insane. But how on earth are we supposed to fix this mess?
2. When you have a segment of society who are actually calling for more restrictions, enforced mask-wearing, etc., it is only a matter of time before we get civilization to collapse.

A. What other conclusions can you draw? It looks like a civilization searching for its own destruction.

January 9, 2022

So is this the end? The ineffable sadness of watching Western civilization walk over the edge of the abyss into nothingness. I guess we had a good three hundred years. As Dowson wrote,

> They are not long, the days of wine and roses:
> Out of a misty dream
> Our path emerges for a while, then closes
> Within a dream.

We keep dreaming this nightmare will end. Omicron seemed to be a gift from God. It is humanized, as Geert and Knut feared, as it can attack those with multiple needles, so no immunity. But amazingly, it is an upper respiratory infection like the common cold, so it is relatively benign and yet confers immunity to the Wuhan virus and its variants. Omicron is, in fact, the ideal vaccine.

So we thought to rejoice. But then, you hear the voices of tyranny. The dear leader of Canada has called those with no, or only a couple of needles, misogynists, and racists. In France, if you don't have boosters, you are a noncitizen, unfit to walk the streets. In Austria, no needles, no shopping for you, and soon, no leaving your home.

So all over the West, the un-needled and un-boosted are unclean, not fit for society. We have heard this before. Soon the jackboots will be heard on the streets and the thunderous knock on the door at night before it is kicked in. Then the transport to the concentration—sorry, quarantine—camps. These have already been built in Australia, and I hear of other places. History does repeat.

With any luck, everyone will get Omicron and then how can the authorities possibly force the needle on everyone? If repeated needling continues, the fear is the immune exhaustion of humans and the immune escape of all viruses. We will know in five to ten years. Maybe the risk is small for us elderly with the weak immune system, but the risk for our children is surely serious.

I never liked Goethe and always thought Young Werther (1774) was an idiot. But I did see one line: "Who rides so late through the night and the storm? It is the father with his child." We hope, we fervently hope, that parents can protect their children from the menace of the needle.

Comment

1. Hopefully, the Supreme Court in the US will rule that mandatory vaccination is unconstitutional.

A. There is hope for the US, but little chance of any such ruling in the rest of the Anglosphere. The courts seem dumb on this issue.

January 14, 2022

Something old, something new! Most of it is not new, just covered up.

Masks. Even CNN now admits that cloth masks do nothing. Any spray painter could have told them that all masks, as currently used en masse, are worse than nothing. Look at the results of the N95 mask in Germany. The horror is that some school boards are forcing children to use an N95. Little kids have a neotenous face with a small nose. Even trained nurses with small noses have a hard time fitting an N95 mask. On a child, it is useless and simply child abuse.

Funding. We knew, almost two years ago, the US Department of Defense refused to fund this "'gain of function'" to humanize a harmless bat virus. But the sainted doctor and his crew funded it anyway. Why? Hubris or something much darker? Put on your tin hat and ask yourself why.

Lockdown. The single biggest disaster in public health history. Everyone except politicians and Public Health Johnnies now know this, and yet, Toronto is on lockdown again. There is no medical reason for this. So why? Schools are closed, further damaging innocent children. This is done, knowing that kids neither get sick nor transmit it. Junior schools in Sweden never closed. So why do it? A deliberate dumbing down of society? Surely not!

Unethical behavior. An email release has shown the unseemly behavior of senior US officials with ad hominem attacks on those who proposed focused protection, which is classic medical teaching upgraded for a highly age-stratified virus.

China is a lockdown success! Well, look again at what is happening in China with cities under lockdown and unwilling inhabitants being forcibly removed to concentration—sorry, quarantine camps. Sadly, the same camps exist in Australia, and rumor has it being built in Canada and New Zealand.

Efficacy of the needle. The CEO of one of the major needle sellers has just admitted that they do very little. So why, oh why, are the politicians so desperate to needle kids with an experimental drug with potential long-term neurological effects?

What's old? In Aldous Huxley's book, *Brave New World*, people lay about doped up with a drug called soma. In my neighborhood, there are now nine new pot shops and precious little else. So who is smoking all that dope? This is an upper-middle-class area where house prices have doubled or tripled in the twenty years I have been here. So this is Zoom, work-at-home territory. So I guess do a Zoom call, do a little work, smoke a lot of dope, look at entertainment, and let the world slide by.

God save us all. Is this the future?

Comment

1. It looks like the future is here. I wonder what those authors of *Brave New World* and *1984* would write today, seeing Earth in its current state of disarray and fear.

A. It looks like what they foresaw was entirely accurate.

January 18, 2022

So Australia, one of the current Omicron hotspots, has deported the tennis star Novak because he is a danger to that country. This action is on par with Canada's senior public health Jenny insisting on the use of face masks during sex and the glee of the follower of Klaus, currently running New Zealand, when she announced concentration—sorry quarantine camps—for the un-needled.

Let us examine the Novak case a little. Currently, no one is allowed onto a plane going to Australia without a valid visa. I know because I once forgot and spent a couple of anxious hours in the LA airport while the people who had invited me to speak there scrambled around to find someone to grant me a temporary visa. I got it, and the temporary visa was good enough for that visit as the plane got into Sydney at midnight. I gave my three talks the next morning and got the same plane back to the US at 3:00 p.m. that afternoon. So Novak had a valid visa. So the revocation was completely arbitrary, a meaningless political show.

Novak had had the virus and recovered. I know that the sainted Dr. F and the CDC have never heard of post-infection immunity. But that's Biology 101, and every doctor in the world knows it exists. Sadly, because of the inexplicable bleating' of the sainted Dr. F, this fact had to be rediscovered about this virus.

Post-infection immunity has been shown to be long-lasting, multivalent, and much more robust than the single valence immunity provided by the needle. That's why further needling with a single valence, when you think of it, is pretty stupid.

That's why, if you have recovered from the virus, the needle is of no value and may actually decrease your multivalent immunity. So Novak posed no risk at all to Australians, needled or not. Anyway, who cares about tennis? I am of an age where I like to see Serena Williams beating the young up-and-comers, but that's about it.

There is good news from the UK. They have just admitted that only a small fraction of the dead actually died of the virus. We knew that, of course, because, in most countries in the world, the excess mortality year on year wasn't much different from 2017 until now, including, believe it or not, the elderly.

So maybe there is the hope of sanity returning. But in Canada, the mandates keep getting worse, and they continue to pursue poor children. We have to resist. Like Kipling's poem:

> When the Horror passing speech
> Hunted us along,
> Each laid hold on each, and each
> Found the other strong.
> In the teeth of Things forbid
> And Reason overthrown.

Comment

1. Wow! Concentration camps. That's something I never thought I would hear in all my days.

A. Me neither. The videos of the camps in Australia and China are terrifying.

January 22, 2022

Dissent, the ability to question and reach a different conclusion, is the basis of Western liberal democracy. If that is fact-checked, de-platformed, and forbidden by politicians, verboten, what society are we living in, and what is worse, what society are we leaving our children?

I have always loathed politicians, but that was because I thought they were self-important, bumbling incompetents. But since the coming of the virus, it has been different. This is beginning to approach Alexander Solzhenitsyn's *Gulag Archipelago* territory. There are already concentration—sorry quarantine camps—in Australia and China. Someone making a perfectly rational medical decision about their own body is now, for unclear reasons, a racist and misogynist, according to the dear leader of Canada.

Why is there this desperation to force everyone into accepting a medical treatment which many don't need and don't want? Israel admits that it has failed, and even the EU is warning against repeated needles. Look it up yourself. I can't say more, as for reasons known only to herself, our Ontario Minister of Health has openly threatened doctors who talk about the needle.

I think we can still talk about other mandates, but I don't know for how long. The mandate police are out in force in Australia and Austria. I find it impossible to believe that it would happen in Canada, but the heroic pastor in Alberta has just been dragged off in chains again and given bellicose statements from our dear leader, the idea sounds not so tin hat anymore.

So what's with this anti-truck driver mandate? These people drive across the continent, usually on their own, but I do have some husband-and-wife teams in my practice. They drive from "point to point", which means that they don't load themselves but pick up and deliver preloaded trailers. So there is minimal person-to-person contact.

Already, when one goes to a food store, there are rows upon rows of empty shelves. What is available often has a startling new price. Inflation is 4 percent, we are told. But not at my gas pump or food store. Surely, even the dear leader of Canada must recognize that if he cancels 20 or 30 percent of truckers, things are going to get really bad. Maybe that is the plan. Sounds crazy, but do you have a better explanation? Is this the new green energy deal in action?

Florida removed all its mandates eighteen months ago and nothing happened. The UK has finally announced that they too will shortly remove all of theirs. That was because their esteemed leader was caught ignoring his own draconian lockdown. So why is Canada still mandating this and that failed policy?

Masking was the silliest of all policies. Thousands, including all spray painters, drywallers, asbestos workers, and anyone who uses a mask at work, knew that it was silly. And yet, it persists, potentially damaging children. The dear leaders at a recent international meeting clearly demonstrate that, for them, it is simply a theatrical prop. So let them carry on with their charade but leave the rest of us to get on with life.

So will this end, or is it simply a prelude to more draconian global warmists' new green lockdowns? Just asking.

Comments

1. It is the same for truck drivers coming into the US from Mexico, which makes even less sense with all the illegals walking across the border with no testing. There is no logical explanation for the mandates. Omicron is everywhere already, so restrictions are useless and destructive.
2. Is this Revelation coming true?

A. I agree. There is no logical explanation or, rather, there is. If you put on your tin hat, this is destabilizing the economies to bring in the Great Reset, which is starting to look like Revelation.

January 28, 2022

Guess what! Naturally acquired immunity exists and is many times stronger, longer lasting, and provides wider immunity to virus variants than a single-valent needle. Eventually, someone has done a study in the US, confirming the Israeli data.

Well, fancy that! Who would have believed that the sainted Dr. F, the CDC, most public health Johnnies, the politicians, and the legacy media would be wrong and that Immunology 101 might be right? The fact of naturally acquired immunity was something every first or second-year medical student knew, but somehow, these "'leaders'" had never heard of it. How could this be? How could anyone ever have taken their statements seriously?

The needle was essentially monovalent, which means it produced immunity to one tiny part of the virus. So all the virus needs is a couple of small mutations, and the needle doesn't work, as the seller has just admitted. Naturally acquired immunity is multivalent, which means that there are antibodies to many areas of the virus, so a small mutation doesn't affect it. That's awfully simplistic, but you get the idea. If you want more details, google "Geert Vanden Bossche."

And despite even the CDC finally admitting what everyone knew, mandates for a needle, which has essentially no effect on the new variants, are still being forced by governments in Canada, Austria, and the like. And they want to needle kids with a substance that does not help and potentially harms them. Why, oh why? Have we returned to the worship of Moloch?

When my coauthor Edna Quammie and I wrote in our book, *The Big House*, about medicine as we knew it decades ago, we traced the rise of political correctness and the gradual elimination of allowable dissent.

If you lose the ability to dissent, you have lost everything. We watched its loss, one silly little step at a time. We never found a hill worth dying on. Now all around us, we see the sorry state we boomers have left. It is hardly an exaggeration to say that it looks like the 1930s with the rise of totalitarianism and collectivism. Who would believe that Australia, New Zealand and increasingly Canada would resemble Germany in the '30s?

In Ontario, Canada, the Minister of Health has openly threatened doctors who talk about the virus with the loss of their medical license. And people wonder why doctors remain passive. It looks like the Enlightenment and freedom are fading away like morning dew.

But maybe there is hope. Driving back the 401 super highway yesterday, the overpasses were crowded with people celebrating the trucker's convoy on its way to Ottawa to face down those intransigent politicians who are destroying the country. Deus Vult or Godspeed these people in their endeavors.

Comment

1. It amazes me how virology 101 was thrown out of the window by the medical establishment complex, all to make people get an experimental needle for profit.

A. In Ontario, if a doctor speaks out, he may lose his license. Hence the profound silence. Something is terribly wrong with this scenario.

February 3, 2022

Bravo to the Canadian truckers. Just when you think all is lost, that the forces hiding behind the curtains are so certain of victory that they are beginning to show themselves, some heroic free men stand up and say, "'Enough'." These heroes are not the effete, ill-educated university class, the Zoom people, or the gray bureaucrats. The truckers are William Tell, Simon Bolivar, and the founders of American freedom.

Funny. I never wanted anything to do with politics. I started these posts because patients and friends were asking what was going on as it all seemed so absurd. Mouthpieces like the sainted Dr. F were making statements that were obviously untrue. Thousands knew them to be untrue, and yet, he stood there in front of the cameras and made them anyway. The bought and paid-for legacy media fawned all over him.

I am just a simple orthopedic surgeon but have a fair research background. I had no interest in immunology or infectious disease. Like the other sheep, I lined up and took whatever needle the authorities suggested. I took the fake needle for the fake H1N1 epidemic. And until last year, I didn't even know it was fake.

I supported Big Pharma because, having been associated with a university all my life, I knew how corrupt and incompetent universities had become, that they had become dominated by bureaucrats, aided by sycophantic has-beens and never-weres.

But these last two years have led me to change my mind, and I simply don't know what to believe anymore. General medical journals have become corrupt to the core. I no longer believe anything the food industry tells me. I think cholesterol is a scam. I now think that a diet should be: increase the protein, reduce the carbs, and if it is manmade, don't eat it.

Two years ago, as I listened to the nonsense being spouted by the sainted Dr. F and his cronies, I thought it was simply because they were just ignorant bureaucrats, and they didn't know any better. But it became progressively more obvious that ignorance and stupidity alone could not explain what was happening.

The denial of naturally acquired immunity was like denying the law of gravity. At that point, it was obvious that this pantomime had nothing to do with a virus. So why and who is pulling the strings of the puppets like our dear leader in Canada? Who do you think?

Let me just return to medicine for a moment. The Toronto school board has just spent two million dollars on face masks for the kids. By now, everyone except the sainted Dr. F, the public health Johnnies and the senior politicians know that face masks on kids is a scam, child abuse. So why? Cui bono? Who is selling these masks? Maybe I am wrong. Maybe it is not corruption but pure and simple ignorance. What do you think?

Comments

1. Follow the money. The PM ordered more boosters, which no one wants, and now the country has to pay. And who benefits?
2. Follow the money. I stopped believing when all the stories conflicted. Who paid for the virus to be developed and why has no one been held responsible? Now three shots don't provide any significant protection and lots of other questions.
3. Definitely corruption. Why are they masking children? Are they trying to produce psychological effects or is it physical? Whatever their reasons, it is not to help the children.
4. Corruption to the core.

A. All these are perfectly valid viewpoints, Occam's razor. What other explanation is there?

February 10, 2022

Here we go again! Take the needle or else! You would think that with the information coming from Israel, which shows the third and fourth needles are not only of no value but, whisper it softly, may damage the immune system, hopefully, temporarily, there would be no more needle mandates. But no. Whoever is in charge of the hospitals has mandated boosters for all.

The operating rooms in many hospitals are closed, not because of too many patients, but because there is no staff. Nurses were fired because they don't want a needle, which has no long-term data on fertility; indeed, no significant data at all.

I thought mandates were coming to an end, but not in Ontario, Canada. Here we remain stout followers of the ever-correct, totally incorruptible independent CDC and the sainted Dr. F. So what to do? Say, "Forget about it," accept hospitals are a lost cause and walk away? Or hang on, obfuscate, and delay? In the UK, the doctors have forced the government to repeal these dreadful mandates of needles for hospital staff, and they have been lifted in all of Scandinavia.

The Canadian feds, led by Justine, the follower of Klaus of Davos, are digging in and planning to pass even more ridiculous mandates blocking interprovincial travel. But there is hope. The valiant truckers have succeeded in forcing some provinces to drop these crazed mandates. But they have been maligned and castigated by the legacy media at the request of the recalcitrant fed. They are being attacked by the bought and paid-for media, police, and agents provocateur. They are standing firm. Think of them, as in the poem:

The song of courage, heart and will,
And gladness in a fight.
Of men who face a hopeless hill,
With sparking and delight.
—Ralph Hodgson, "The Song of Honour"

Deus Vult! They will win against the hosts of darkness. But even if they fail, the eyes of the world are on them. And they can tell their kids, as did Henry the Fifth before the battle of Agincourt,

We few, we happy few, we band of brothers;
For he to-day that stands with me
Shall be my brother.

—*Henry V*

When I started writing about this virus two years ago, the issues were medical. But that soon went away, and by May 2020, we realized that whatever was happening, it had nothing to do with medicine or a virus. That was hard to accept. Initially, I thought Occam's razor, that the explanation of the unthinkable was stupidity, as the public health Johnnies are notoriously not the sharpest nails in the medical box. These people in charge, the "top docs" as the legacy media call them, are really not doctors at all but simply bureaucrats.

It is hard to think of a time-serving bureaucrat leading a vast conspiracy. But then, it was just such bureaucrats, the Adolf Eichmann's, acting under orders, who kept the trains running to Auschwitz when the German military was collapsing around them. So when will this madness end? Or is this just the beginning?

Comments

1. After what I went through after the second shot, they will have to tie me down for any more.
2. I had the stupid needle three times. Ruined the use of my hands.

A. The problem is the vast underreporting of the complications of the needle. Such reporting is, I am told, difficult, time-consuming, and discouraging. So we don't know what the complications are and the frequency.

February 15, 2022

Just published a new book, *Plague or Pseudo Plague 2021.* My concern is that electronic history will be edited to conform to the new ruler's perception of reality, and I thus wanted a permanent record of what actually happened. I was not sure the lawyers would allow publication. As I expected, they did insist on significant editing for fear of retribution from the mandate fanatics.

We now think that the virus escaped from the Wuhan lab in May of 2019. It was likely deliberately spread during the Military World Games in Wuhan in October of 2019. With the connivance of WHO, it was certainly broadcast all over the world during Chinese New Year when internal flights were banned but international flights from Wuhan continued all over the world, including three flights a week into Northern Italy.

It would normally just have been a bad flu year, nothing special, but what happened was inexplicable. The lockdown was a concept never considered in the West. And yet, with the help of WHO, the Imperial College shill, the professor doctor who amped up the PCR test, and the sainted Dr. F, this CCP-induced disaster was initiated in Italy and then enforced all over the world. The West committed collective economic and cultural suicide. A generation of children was damaged.

It should have been clear to even the dullest scientist or medic by May 2020 that the lockdown was a failure and the collateral damage immense. And yet it continued, we thought because of the desire to unseat the US incumbent and in other places, like France, to quell the dissatisfaction and riots over the green energy policy failures.

I published my 2020 posts in book form, *Journal of the Plague Year (2020)*, as history was being edited, and I wanted to leave an accurate account. I never thought that the craziness would continue for a further year, and yet here we are, book two, *Plague or Pseudo Plague 2021*.

In spite of the shining examples of Florida and Sweden, the useless mandates continue, and in Canada, martial law has been declared. So we have no idea where this will end.

As before, this new book contains my largely unedited posts of last year with many of my readers' acerbic and amusing comments. Some have been heavily edited by the publisher's lawyers in spite of the fact that they survived the FB fact-checkers. So censorship is alive and well.

Comment

1. And so it continues. So many blind, deaf, and uniformed followers of the legacy media. The frightening question is when will it stop, if ever?

A. Klaus of Davos believes this is a great opportunity to change the world with his Great Reset. If he succeeds, it will never end.

February 17, 2022

What is going on? The recent actions by federal governments in some countries show clearly that their actions have nothing to do with a none-too-serious virus.

All the working guys in the Canadian trucker convoy are asking is that mandates which make no sense be revoked. Let us examine some of them.

Needle passports. As the needle neither stops infection nor its transmission, the passport serves no purpose.

Boosters or any needle for the healthy. As Israel has shown, repeated boosters do not stop infection or hospitalization. Omicron actually is the best vaccine, being highly infectious and with very low morbidity.

Border transit. North America is a big continent with widespread virus dissemination. To allow East/West passage and block North/South makes no sense.

Lockdown. It has been repeatedly shown to have no positive effects and has huge collateral damage.

Tracing apps on phones. Test and trace were never possible with a high-infection, low-morbidity airborne virus. So they serve no medical purpose.

I was listening to the traffic reports on the car radio this morning and was shocked by the poisonous hatred of the truckers' protest being spewed out by the radio announcer and his guests. The level of vitriol was incomprehensible. But I see the same on any legacy media channel. Where does this hate come from?

I grew up in a small mining village in Scotland. I went to university while my boyhood friends went down the mines. As a doctor working in the Canadian state system, more than half of all my patients were and are working class. I liked them as a boy, and I like them now. To listen to these ill-educated, pompous, none-too-bright members of the Zoom class slandering those honorable working guys was very disconcerting.

There seems to be a working-class uprising all over the world about these foolish, crippling, worthless mandates imposed by the collectivist bureaucracy. Given the inexplicable resistance by governments to these common-sense requests, God alone knows how this will end.

Comments

1. I would rather die on my feet than live on my knees.
2. This is a nightmare for Canadians. All we wanted was for the vaccine passports gone and for the people who were fired to get their jobs back. And now the Liberal government has, in effect, declared martial law.
3. The federal gang is semi-orgasmic, watching the arrests under the Emergency Measures Act. It has become a police state, not my country.

A. It is hard to recognize this as the country I came to fifty years ago.

February 24, 2022

God be praised! The truckers have won. The dear leader of Canada and follower of Klaus has rescinded martial law.

But did the truckers really win? One is tempted to rejoice, but was this merely one step back in preparation for two steps forward? Let us look soberly at what is actually happening.

One of the lady organizers of this peaceful protest, a Métis grandmother, is still in jail with no bail in Canada for a crime of misdemeanor!

Mandates. Some of the provinces of Canada had dropped them, but the feds continue. This is in spite of the fact that all mandates have been repeatedly shown to be of no medical value and some have had catastrophic effects. Clearly, these mandates have nothing to do with infectious disease. So why continue? Omicron is an upper respiratory infection like the common cold. It is seasonal, endemic, and will not go away.

I am no lawyer, but clearly, if a minority government can bring in martial law and survive a vote of nonconfidence, then what is to stop them from reintroducing it next week or next year because of some fantasy crisis like global warming? If it can be justified for a few trucks parked in Ottawa, then what? When will there be a fire in the Reichstag like in Berlin in 1933? No Western leader openly rebuked the imposition of martial law in Canada. So now that it is clear it can be done in a Western country with no blowback, which country will be next? Two years ago, who would have believed that?

Child abuse. We have known for two years that kids were at no risk, they neither got seriously ill nor transmitted the virus. What they have been subjected to is inconceivable with two years of lockdown. They are behind in education and some will never catch up. The smaller kids are behind in speech, and who knows what psychological damage has been done by the failure of socialization. They are certainly depressed and fearful, but what else? What damage has isolation done to their immunity, even if they are not forced to accept the needle? This is called the hygiene hypothesis. If kids are not exposed to a wide array of viruses, they do not develop adequate immunity. So we can expect to see large outbreaks, probably of the respiratory syncytial virus, next winter.

And what is happening with the Canadian banks? Does the dear leader still have the ability to block people's access to their own money? I have no idea.

So, sadly, it looks as if the Western world is a very different place than it was a week ago. Is this the end of the Enlightenment? Are we looking at a collectivist nightmare, *Brave New World* and *1984*? This can't be real. It must be a bad dream.

We hope so, but I tremble for the world we are leaving our children.

March 1, 2022

How bad will it get? I just heard the words, “pure blood,” used by a clever woman in an interview. That echo of the ’30s sends a shiver down the spine. What was worse was that she talked about organ harvesting.

Sounds crazy, a true tin-hat lunacy. But she was describing recent work from Sweden, which showed that the RNA from the needle gets rapidly incorporated into human DNA in liver cells. What then?

If it does what we believe it is supposed to do, it will produce the spike protein, and the body will destroy its own liver. Will this actually happen in real life as opposed to a cell culture? Who knows? I have been hearing for months about the spike protein migrating up the vagus nerve. That seemed so wildly fantastical I could not believe it. But, but, if it is even remotely a little bit true, then Mary, Mother of God, protect us.

Even if it is only a psychotic nightmare with no basis in reality, at least, protect the children until it can be disproved by animal studies. Once the needle mRNA products are in the body, you can’t get them out. If they become part of human DNA, then we have the two classes of humans the woman was talking about.

If the Swedish study scales up from the laboratory, then life for the needled will be as Hobbes described, “Nasty, brutish, and short.” If there is widespread liver failure, the only treatment is a transplant. And the new liver would have to come from a non-needled person. Hence her talk about organ harvesting.

This will never happen in the West. We don’t have quarantine camps. Oh, but we do! And in Xinjiang, there are whispers of organs for sale. In the West, we couldn’t force people into these camps. We don’t have the authority. Oops! In Canada, NZ, and Australia, we did, and the rest of the world said nothing.

No! I am sure that this is a waking nightmare brought on by the lockdown. People are afraid because of the fear porn produced by the legacy media, loneliness, depression, inflation, job loss, poverty, and despair. I am sure everything will be A-OK, and everyone will be just fine. I hope. I really hope so.

Comment

1. Those of us who refused the needle will be watching intently. I sincerely hope you are wrong, but then, they did mandate a needle of unknown toxicity and very little evidence of value.

A. We all hope that it will never come to this.

March 6, 2022

Just when you think things are returning to normal, another piece of idiocy pops up. The competitors in the Iditarod have to be needled. Ye gods and little fishes! Sick people don't run the Iditarod, the one-thousand-mile dog sled race from Anchorage to Nome, which usually takes about nine days. These incredibly fit men have to be needled. Maybe their dogs also!

Surely by now even the dullest public health Johnny knows that even the CDC has admitted that the needle neither stops infection nor transmission. Indeed, looking at Israel, it seems the more boosters, the sicker the population.

We would expect lunacy like this from Australia where the world's greatest tennis player, who had recovered from the virus and therefore had strong natural immunity, was not allowed to play unless he got a totally counterproductive needle. Similar idiocy would be expected from the followers of Klaus of Davos running New Zealand and Canada, but the last time I looked, Alaska was part of the US.

As a boy growing up in Scotland, I knew nothing about America other than TV Westerns. *Cooper's Last of the Mohicans* was popular, but Jack London's books, *Call of the Wild* and *White Fang*, about Alaska and the Yukon were so memorable. Hard to think of these people taking a needle for effectively the common cold.

Robert Service's poems about that harsh environment were unforgettable:

> Have you know the Great White Silence
> not a snow gemmed twig aquiver?

Or his great poem about the Yukon working girl:

> Was I not born to walk in scorn where others walk in pride?
> The Maker marred, and, evil starred, I drift upon His tide;
> But He alone shall judge His own,
> so I His judgment bide.

I used that phrase to describe one of the main characters in my five-volume series, *To Slip the Surly Bonds of Earth*, now finally all in audiobooks.

In Canada, we still have a lady in prison who helped organize the truckers' protest. I am no lawyer, but to refuse bail for a charge of a misdemeanor is hard to understand, almost Kafkaesque. Is this revenge because our dear leader of Canada was afraid of the truckers and ran off and hid until he could bring in martial law on a peaceful protest?

Silly me. I thought I lived in a country where there was a rule of law.

Comment

1. Apparently, no one is reading the nine pages of complications of the needle. Profits reign supreme and the mass media is bought and sold. So many conspirators and so little curiosity.

A. Other than a few heroes like the truckers, it is almost a universal collective brainwash.

March 13, 2022

Look back in anger! A world destroyed. Kids were effectively jailed for two years; the petite bourgeoisie, the lower middle class, and the backbone of a functioning nation were deliberately ruined; cheap reliable energy was deliberately disrupted and priced out of reach; roaring inflation wiped out savings; an experimental drug injected into half the world. Why? Were these actions of the oligarchs, the ruling elite, deliberately destructive or due to hubris and stupidity?

Maybe it is simply that all civilizations contain telomeres, the death genes present in all life-forms. The rise and fall of empires are well documented. Eternal Rome collapsed because the currency was debased: the lower class did no work being supported by welfare, bread, and circuses. The ruling class lost all sense of integrity and honesty. Sounds familiar, eh?

China has seen five such empires and has described the cycle, which is always the same. First is the rise of the hero, who comes out of chaos and establishes order and the rule of law. Then there is the golden age where everything flourishes. People believe in honesty, courage, patriotism, and the dignity of the family. Next is the merchant age when currency is debased, debt rises, and real wages decline. Honesty and morality are seen as old-fashioned and mocked. Then ensues the age of chaos when everything collapses. The only grim satisfaction is that the elites, responsible for this tragedy, never survive.

In the West, we have seen this with the collapse of the empires of Greece, Rome, Byzantium, Spain, and Britain. The Western explanation is similar to China, that bad times produce strong men. Strong men produce good times. Good times produce weak men, and weak men produce bad times. How true!

Can the West recover or is the Enlightenment over? Sadly it seems that we are well along the scenario described by Hayek in 1944 in his book, *The Road to Serfdom.*

As a surgeon, I had no interest in politics. But this is not the wide-open, sky's-the-limit Canada I came to in 1971. It was wonderful, full of "the roaring boys' bravado." But then, it all seeped away. And now we have martial law because the truckers, the working people I admire, dared to peacefully protest about insane and unscientific mandates.

We older people are stuck. But where should our kids go to look for freedom in an unfree world?

Comments

1. Back in '72, even with the first Trudeau's stupid fiscal policies and resulting inflation, society still ran on principles and work ethics, and it functioned well. We expected it to get better. Don't you wish the adults were still in charge?
2. It is not so bad here in the US, as we are a union of states, and some have stayed free and defied the federal government. I am confident that "we the people" will win.

A. One lives in hope. Kristi Noem in South Dakota is a shining example of what is possible, as is Ron DeSantis in Florida.

March 19, 2022

Guess what I heard! The virus was an "incapacitating agent." Now it begins to make sense.

There was much about the virus which was unusual. It had an unbelievable age gradient. The risk of death to the healthy under sixty was almost negligible and rose steeply after seventy. The majority of deaths were in people long after retirement age, and most actually over normal life expectancy.

Ockham's razor suggests that the simplest explanation is the correct one. So I assumed that the virus had been manufactured to eliminate the unproductive elderly on pensions, which increasingly governments could not afford as so-called government retirement pensions were actually a giant Ponzi scheme. However, if the excess mortality year over year and country over the country is examined, there is nothing, nothing at all. There was no lethal epidemic. So the virus failed. So maybe that wasn't the objective after all.

I recently heard a persuasive argument that it was a bioweapon, but not a lethal one, instead an incapacitating agent. A tin hat theory maybe, but it makes sense. It is airborne, highly infectious, and readily transmissible. It simply makes people sick for a few days.

Imagine if it were deployed by drones over Taiwan. The military gets sick, and you walk in with no fighting, no deaths, and no destruction of facilities. Fait accompli! Perfect! But to do so, you would need a needle to give your own troops immunity for a few months. Rumor is that such a needle was in development in 2018. So the virus' escape in May 2019 was about two years ahead of schedule.

Once the genie was out of the bottle in Wuhan in May 2019, what to do? Maybe move to plan B. Maybe the CCP, the WEF, and Big Pharma saw an opportunity to advance whatever plans they had. By creating alarm and confusion, destroy the economy of the West, the middle class, and eliminate the wretched of the earth, those living hand-to-mouth; by starvation, malaria, TB, etc.? And sell vast quantities of needles with no long-term data, minimal animal testing, and under the guise of an emergency with no legal ramifications.

But that still begs the question of why Sweden, Brazil, and I think Belarus, follow centuries of Western medicine. Why did the public health Johnnies and the politicians in all other countries follow the CCP? One can see the influence of WEF in countries like Canada and others, and maybe Big Pharma money. Why were Western medicine and common sense kicked out the door, and cheap, effective drugs banned? Even discussion was banned, and docs were threatened with loss of medical license if they discussed the needle, something which had never been done before.

Stupidity is a convenient explanation. But is it the right one? What do you think?

Comments

1. It was pretty obvious early on that this was a plandemic, and the motives might be many. We thought initially it was to remove Trump from office. I am an expert in respiratory protection, so I knew immediately when they started with the masks that it was all phony.
2. Many questions, no answers. And there won't be any. Too much profit in keeping the answers hidden.

A. Sadly so.

April 6, 2022

"*Fuit Ilium*" (Troy was) as Virgil wrote in 40 BC. When I was a boy, we knew all about Troy. One recent poet wrote,

> Who would remember Helen,
> were she not surrounded by spears.

But that is misreading history. It is the opposite; who would remember Troy were it not for Helen? Another poet described her:

> Was this the face that launch'd a thousand ships
> And burnt the topless towers of Ilium?"
> --Christopher Marlowe, *Dr. Faustus.*

Ilium or Troy fell to the Greeks, then the Greeks to Rome, and even Rome, the eternal city, fell in 400 AD, ushering in one thousand years of despair, darkness, and savagery.

Currently, we look at the disaster all around, a world crumbling into ruins, sliding into a manufactured totally unnecessary nuclear war.

The global warmists have destroyed cheap and reliable energy such that Canada and the US, sitting on lakes of oil, have to import this essential ingredient of modern civilization from potentially hostile countries. Europe destroyed its domestic energy production and is dependent on Russia, on whom it has effectively and nonsensically declared war.

The futile war has reduced supplies of grain and fertilizer such that starvation in some parts of the world is a real issue. Inflation is reaching record highs, and yet, those nominally in charge continue to print worthless money with gay abandon. I guess they have never heard of Venezuela, Argentina, and the Weimar Republic.

To think that, as little as three years ago, the world looked forward to endless prosperity. It certainly was not ideal as the forces of malignancy, the Frankfurt school of Antonio Gramsci and Adorno had largely destroyed Western public education, the legacy media, and entertainment.

We look back a few years and dream of a time, as Tacitus (AD 90) described when you could "think what you like and say what you think." But even in the '70s and '80s, that was slipping away, as Edna Quammie and I documented in our book, *The Big House*, a lighthearted memoir of the wild and wonderful times in Toronto General when it was one of the world's great hospitals. Even then, we could see the dead hand of political correctness slithering in.

So what happened in the last three years? I was always taught to assume stupidity before malevolence. But the tragedy has been so great that stupidity alone is not an excuse. The virus? Well, when you look at the excess mortality rates year on year and country over country, where was this epidemic? It's hard to find.

What is tragic is the demographics of those who died; unexpectedly, it is the young. And they didn't die of any virus. Lockdown and possibly some "treatments" look like the cause. But in spite of Elon Musk's move into social media, we remain under the control of fierce algorithms and, therefore, have to moderate our statements. Doctors cannot comment on the needle in any meaningful way, as if they do, they may lose their medical license.

So where will it end? There is no sign of sanity returning. Kids remain masked for a disease that never affected them and which they never transmitted. In spite of the abject lesson of Israel, the needle is still being pushed hard. The health care system, at least in Canada, remains in total disarray. With hyperinflation, energy and food shortages, and the war on the horizon, what to do? There is no safe place.

I guess we struggle on, putting one foot in front of the other, on the way to Golgotha. Deus Vult! Tomorrow is another day.

Comments

1. Given the success of the mRNA needle, ha, ha, when will they start to push a full spectrum needle which will cure all illnesses?

2. They are now offering shot number four. If it didn't work the last time, let's do it again.

1A. That is the worry. If they can get away with mandating a gene therapy as "effective" when it has really not been tested and has many side effects, when will they start to sell the world a cure-all needle which will "work'" on rhinoviruses and other common cold viruses? Such a move could well be a disaster and wipe out the human race.

2A. Hope springs eternal in the breast of the bureaucrat. They are like the WWI generals: "Just run into the machine guns again boys. This time it will be different."

April 13, 2022

I saw three kids in my medical clinic the other day with aches and pains here and there. And no, they had not had the needle recently, which is the first thing I ask patients with unexplained pains, rashes, and in particular, neurological problems. So what's the diagnosis?

It is the collateral damage of the lockdown. I am seeing this all the time now. Kids with back pain as they sit hunched over their computer or cell phone for hours on end. After a gap of two years, the kids are out, playing sports. So they are sore from the unaccustomed activity.

Don't blame the kids. In Canada, for two years, they have been denied their youth, effectively jailed in solitary confinement; no friends, no school, no sports; and a constant barrage of lies and fear porn. And now they come out, blinking in the sunshine. As Francis Thompson wrote,

> I stand amid the dust of the mounded years—
> My mangled youth lies dead beneath the heap.
> My days have crackled and gone up in smoke,
> Have puffed and burst as sun-starts in a stream.
>
> —"The Hound of Heaven"

Unthinking, uncaring bureaucrats did this to them. We knew by May 2020 that the lockdown was a disaster and that kids neither got sick nor transmitted the virus. We knew from the results in Sweden that junior school closures were unnecessary. And yet, the voices of reason, those who dared point this out were silenced.

I avoided the worst of the censorship by publishing in book form. If interested, google my books, *Journal of the Plague Year* (2020) and *Plague or Pseudo Plague 2021.*

Surrounded by this constant drumbeat of fear, no wonder the kids are emotionally damaged. So don't be surprised. And don't blame them for their fears and timidity. Don't blame the victims.

I don't find physiotherapy of any value to these kids as it is too medicalized. The girls I send to dance class—if young, to ballet, and if older, to jazz or hip hop. The boys I send to basketball. I find the coaches and instructors in these disciplines just great with kids. They keep pushing them, and it gives them poise, balance, and confidence.

The other problem is the parents. They may have lost their job or their business because of the lockdown. They may have been fired because of these insane mandates. They are looking at financial ruin, and with inflation roaring on, they see that they will lose their homes as well. It is hard for a stressed-out parent to listen to a whining child.

The next decade will be really tough with runaway inflation. We older people remember the Jimmy Carter years, but the young have never known it. What seems also to be happening is the increase in censorship. The Canadian federal government wishes to control social media so that only the official view is allowed. So posts like this may be deemed disruptive and banned. Three short years ago, who would have imagined a world like this?

Comments

1. So many are blinded in denial of reality.
2. I hope Canadians will decide at some stage to stand up to the dictatorship.

A. We hope but how? The politicians and legacy media all sing the same tune, as do schools and universities, licensing authorities, and increasingly big business.

April 21, 2022

Sanity at last! A US judge has finally struck down the mask mandates for planes. Sadly, in Toronto, masking continues in many venues, including clinics, hospitals, grocery stores, etc.

Why this should be remains unclear. Universal masking had no scientific basis. Everyone who knew anything about masking knew that including even the sainted Dr. F before he began to shill for one, then two, then three masks. The obvious reason for his change of direction was to increase the drumbeat of fear to force the mandatory needling of those who neither needed it nor wanted it.

If anyone needs an education on masking, they should ask their neighborhood spray painter, drywaller, or asbestos worker if they would use a surgical or even an N95 mask for work. When they stop laughing, they will explain particle size. Forget clinical trials. Thousands of people all over the world, certainly most of the skilled trades, knew that universal masking was a joke and a hoax.

Surgeons wear masks in the OR to stop drooling into the wound and to protect themselves from blood splash. I believe that there is actually no evidence that surgical masks reduce the incidence of wound infection. The only time we surgeons use face shields like a welder's shield is when we are using power tools and the patient has something like hepatitis C or AIDS. It probably doesn't help, but blood splash from these cases frightens the surgeon.

The masking of little kids was simply child abuse and virtually only done in North America. Even the despicable WHO condemned it, and it was never done in Europe. It was not only ineffective and silly, but it was harmful to the children, both psychologically and in terms of development. Whether or not they will ever catch up remains to be seen.

The health care system in Canada remains a disaster area with waiting lists stretching out into infinity. I hear the UK is just as bad. I don't know about anywhere else. Will it ever return to normal? I have grave doubts. Examinations of medical students for the last two years have been done through Zoom. The authorities in Ontario are so far behind in the licensing examinations of doctors from other countries that I read that they are dropping the exams. I hope I misread that.

The constant yammer of mandatory needling for everyone, including little kids, seems a little muted recently. It should be, considering the results from Israel. Boosters don't seem to help anything and are possibly confirming the worst fears of Geert and Knut. The mention of the fears of these eminent scientists is never reported by the legacy media. As Goethe said, "Excellence is rarely found and rarely valued."

For fear of the fierce algorithm, one cannot say more. Sadly, the voices of misinformation from authorities like the CDC continue. As Montaigne said, "The world has never lacked for charlatans."

Comments

1. Every time I see the word, "expert," in a post or article, I feel like throwing the damn phone across the room. The past two years have not been science at its finest.
2. The dear leader of Canada has done such an abysmal job, it is difficult to credit. The truckers were right about needle mandates, which are increasingly being shown to be of no value whatsoever.

1A. As soon as a qualifier is added, like "the" science, it changes it. "The" science is not science, it is Faucian logic. Like "social" justice, which has nothing to do with justice.

2A. The results from Israel and Gaza certainly show that the truckers were right; and the CDC, the sainted Dr. F, the public health Johnnies, and politicians were wrong.

April 29, 2022

The sun is shining on the way to work! After a long Canadian winter, it makes you think of Kipling's poem, "The Flowers":

> Robin down the logging-road whistles, "Come to me!"
> Spring has found the maple-grove, the sap is running free;
> All the winds of Canada call the plowing-rain,
> Take the flower and turn the hour, and kiss your love again.

I will never forget when I came to Canada in 1971—the vibrancy, the wildness bursting with life, a new world, new ideas, and a future with years that never end and know no sorrow. The wonder of it will live in my memory forever.

And then the medical clinic fills up: achy people, the depressed, those who lost their business, losing their house. Some of their aches are just a physical manifestation of their psychic distress. And the poor kids, still wearing these ridiculous paper masks! Surely, by now, everyone, except the sainted Dr. F and the CDC, knows that universal masking was a joke and a hoax.

Someone made money out of selling all that worthless PPE, including that Plexiglas, which still surrounds everything. A moment's thought would make it obvious that a Plexiglas barrier will reduce airflow, and so, increases the likelihood of airborne infection. It does not decrease it.

And we still have these frantic exhortations to wash our hands, which has no effect on an airborne virus. Or rather, maybe it has.

The hygiene hypothesis is that if little kids are kept too clean, they will not develop proper immunity. The increased incidence of respiratory syncytial virus and the even more deadly childhood hepatitis, which is currently rampant in the UK, suggests that the hypothesis is real. And what effect the additional needle will have? No one knows.

One is still afraid to mention the needle, which, in spite of the obvious failure in Israel, is still being pushed on kids. The various Quangos, quasi-autonomous nongovernment organizations, still threaten docs who dare question the party line.

Surrounded by rampant inflation and dire warnings of food shortages to come, one is amazed at how many food processing plants in the US are burning down.

Is Shanghai the future with hungry people locked in apartment buildings? Is this the Great Reset trumpeted by so many Western leaders? The fact that martial law could be declared in Canada with virtually no protests hardly gives confidence in the future of democracy. Will the kids, who have never known anything but authoritarianism, accept such a dystopian world?

Quel dommage! What a pity! Maybe a walk in the sunshine will make the world seem a better place.

Comments

1. In our post office, they have finally taken down these plastic walls.
2. The sun always makes one feel hope, even though it is always followed by darkness. I see in Denmark they are not going to give any more needles.

A. Some signs of sanity returning. These Plexiglas walls were the height of lunacy. They are still all over the place in hospitals, and I doubt that they will ever be removed. Similarly, I think that these silly mask rules are here to stay in hospitals. The news from Denmark is great. No more needles for the young. It would be too much to hope for such sanity in Canada.

May 8, 2022

Spring has sprung, the grass is riz,
I wonder where the flowers is.

In Canada, we know that finally, it is spring because the magnificent magnolia trees are in bloom everywhere.

Not quite as good as Japan. I remember being on the grounds of Hirosaki Castle when the magnolias and the Sakura were blooming at the same time. I have always thought that the Sakura, the short-lived cherry blossoms, symbolized the fleeting beauty of life. As Burns wrote,

Like the snow falls in the river,
A moment white—then melts forever;
Or like the borealis race,
That flit ere you can point the place.
—"Tam o' Shanter"

And then sadly, you listen to social media where the information about the harsh reality of the worst public health disaster in history is coming out, trickling around the dams erected by the censors.

The actual figures are available, buried in the morass of statistics being twisted by the sleazy and skillful spinmeisters of the legacy media. It is now generally acknowledged, except by the CDC and the sainted Dr. F, that the lockdown was responsible for almost triple the deaths directly due to the virus. The exact figures don't matter, only that the "cure" was infinitely worse than the disease. And we knew this by the spring of 2020.

The full extent of the tragedy is only beginning. We have always known that poverty and despair lead to spikes in the reduction of life expectancy and the increase in death rates. And yet the self-proclaimed public health "experts" ignored these known facts and forced this pointless and catastrophic lockdown, similar to that being imposed currently in Shanghai.

The long-term effects on children will be generational. Kids were deprived, terrified, and brutalized for a disease that never affected them. The junior schools in Sweden never closed, and yet, no teacher was ever infected by a student.

The lunacy continues with various mandates in spite of the worst fears of Geert and Knut coming true. Reduced immunity appears real, and the more the needles, the worse the effects with the reactivation of dormant DNA viruses like Epstein-Barr and shingles. How far this acquired immune deficiency syndrome, or AIDS, to give it its name, will go remains to be seen. At least, this time, the sainted Dr. F is not pushing AZT on them although the one that is being pushed may turn out to be no better.

Even more tragically, many so-called "leaders" appear to be using *1984* and *Brave New World* as a blueprint, rather than a cautionary tale. The US and Canada seem to be introducing the Ministry of Truth, their truth, and none other.

Was this none-too-serious virus the cause or just a convenient excuse for the changes occurring? Who knows! What do you think?

Comment

1. Will the truth about the disastrous mishandling of this outbreak ever be told? Money and power can rewrite anything.

A. And those most affected by this plot or lunacy have none.

May 14, 2022

"The owl of Minerva spreads its wings only with the coming of the dusk," wrote Hegel, meaning that wisdom is only achieved in hindsight. Some of these tragedies we are beginning to wake up to, and some remain hidden in the next week or month or year.

Hindsight makes it clear to us that the world has just experienced and continues to experience the worst public health disaster in history.

This began with the insanity of "gain of function" research, making a harmless animal virus infect humans, thus creating a bioweapon. Lab leaks occur even in the best level 4 labs, but to fund and carry out such research in the known leaky CCP military-run lab in a country not exactly the friend of the West is hard to understand. A Benedict Arnold moment? No one has paid any price for this. So is it continuing?

We now suspect the virus was out in the spring of 2019, and certainly, spread during the International Military Games in Wuhan in the fall of 2019. As a conference was held in New York in the fall of 2019, entitled Event 201, discussing measures to be taken around a coronavirus epidemic, you don't need much of a tin hat to believe that people knew what was coming long before the widespread virus triggered seasonally.

Initially, we thought that this was the Big One, the Spanish flu or the Black Death. But then the *Diamond Princess* cruise ship showed that it was very tightly targeted at the ill elderly and some with other comorbidities. And yet knowing this, the world lockdown took place. Unnecessary, futile, and wickedly destructive. It has been responsible already for far more deaths than the virus.

The lockdown was based on designating people who tested positive "cases," sick or not! Based on the PCR test, which the developer, Kary

Mullis, said was never to be used as a diagnostic tool. Similarly, fear was whipped up by calling all deaths "from" the virus when about 90 percent were simply "with."

Incredibly, repositioned drugs were demonized or frankly banned for no clear reason. The needle, which rumor has it, was available two years prior——. I had better say no more. Docs in Canada lose their medical license for discussing the needle. If interested, google "Geert and Knut."

Now that the fear of the virus is receding, we see around us economic collapse with soaring inflation and food shortages. Food shortages! No baby formula? In the developed world! How could this happen? And soaring costs of energy because our dear leaders in the West refuse to extract from the vast oil reserves we are sitting on.

Why this death wish? The original Pope Benedict, an optimist, said, "Pruned, it grows again." Augustine, the Bishop of Hippo, looking across the Mediterranean at the lights going out in Rome, said, "It is finished." And it was. The lights remained out for a thousand years of the Dark Ages. Is this what we are looking at? Are our "leaders" leading us over the edge of the abyss? Why? What do you think?

Comment

1. It seems clear that the elite plan on ruling. A numerically reduced and fearful populace dependent on rulers for food and shelter is easier to control. Agenda 21 in action.

May 16, 2022

Tomorrow, and tomorrow, and tomorrow,
Creeps in this petty pace from day to day.

—*Macbeth*

I was in a restaurant yesterday for only the second time since the start of the virus disaster. It was a reasonably rated Thai restaurant, and since I first went to Thailand, I have always liked everything Thai. Their surgeons were so good that the amount of teaching I did there was unfortunately limited to two or three occasions only.

I don't drink anymore, so I have no idea what beer costs in most places, but $9 for a small bottle? Eh? This strikes me as real inflation. The vegetarian food was excellent, but $19 for fried plantain and a dipping sauce seems excessive. The beef, sadly, was not so good. Got to cut back somewhere, I guess.

What amazed me was that even at these prices, the place was full of young people. This was Thai, not French, but even so, how could they afford it?

My young son, in his early twenties, thought it was because many in his generation have given up on savings. There is no chance that they will ever be able to buy a house in Toronto or any major city. With soaring inflation, spurred on by reckless politicians printing money by the billions and shipping it out into the great unknown with no oversight and no checks or balances, what is the point in saving? The money will be worthless tomorrow or the next day, so eat, drink, be merry, and ignore tomorrow. The young people see this as a replay of Argentina or Venezuela or the Weimar Republic.

I try to avoid the news, having given up on legacy media years ago as what they report usually bears no relation to the truth. Even formerly reputable medical journals are so woke that they are not worth reading. But everywhere I turn, I hear rumors of disaster, that countries are going to turn over sovereignty to that utterly corrupt and worthless WHO.

In the dark night of the soul, I wonder if this is a replay of Europe in the '30s, stumbling into WWII. Intolerable conditions lead to revolts which produce Napoleons or worse. As the poem about Napoleon goes,

> "How far is St. Helena from a fight in Paris street?"
> I haven't time to answer now—the men are falling fast.
> The guns begin to thunder, and the drums begin to beat.
> (*If you take the first step, you will take the last.*)
>
> —"A St. Helena Lullaby"

Deus Vult, I hope not. The rain has stopped, and the sun is shining. Time to go out and walk and dream of a better world.

Comment

1. Seniors can dream, middle age can hope, the young—is there anything for them but despair?

A. How true and how sad. How different from when we were young, "in the glad morning of our day."

May 20, 2022

> "Oh judgment thou art fled to brutish beasts,
> And men have lost their reason"
> (*Julius Caesar*, Act 3, Scene 2).

Have you heard? The West is about to sign over authority to WHO. If our dear leaders sign this document, the director of WHO can unilaterally declare a pandemic and order whatever he thinks fits. Given the actual numbers who died of the virus as opposed to dying with, and most according to the very suspect PCR test, any flu year, or indeed anything can be called a pandemic. They have changed the wording of what used to be a pandemic, removing the word, "lethal."

One may wish to remember that the current head of WHO, who calls himself a doctor but isn't, is actually a Marxist and owes his position to President Xi. He was the one who claimed that person-to-person infection did not occur; claimed that flights from Wuhan were safe; helped institute that disastrous, and unscientific lockdown and universal crazy masking.

One recognizes that several of our dear leaders believe that the countries they have been elected to run are post-national, and so are glad to cede power to a one-world government run possibly by Klaus of Davos and his think-alikes. It is hard to imagine anything worse.

And we have this new monkeypox, or as someone called it, money pox. I hear it is difficult to catch and not terribly lethal. But it is being touted as requiring smallpox vaccination and quarantine. I guess most people have given up being scared of the Faucian virus, so time for a new one.

Increasingly, it sounds like Salman Rushdie's 2019 book, *Quichotte*, where the world collapses into insanity and another dimension. I guess you don't know what freedom is until you lose it. Boethius, AD 520, wrote that "the bitterest part is to remember you were happy once." He also wrote that "the worst of times, like the best, are always passing away," except his worst of times, the Dark Ages, lasted one thousand years.

Our poor kids have never known freedom so maybe they won't miss it. So for the rest of us, I guess, "eat, drink and be merry for tomorrow we die." Or read my favorite poem, the *Rubáiyát*,

> Ah, make the most of what we yet may spend,
> Before we too into the Dust descend.

We are after all,

> Like Snow upon the Desert's dusty Face
> Lighting a little Hour or two—is gone.

I suppose we should hope. As Scarlet O'Hara said, "Tomorrow is another day."

Comments

1. For those of us who are older, we see mandates and other changes with alarm. My son, age thirty-three, thinks I am being too negative about governments and the Great Reset. I tell him I am alarmed about his and my grandchildren's future.
2. America still has a vast number of armed citizens. Admiral Yamamoto said, "I fear all we have done is awaken the sleeping giant and fill him with a terrible resolve."

A. I hope. I really hope that the sleeping giant will awaken, as the US is the world's last best hope. Sadly, there is little sign of it. I hope it is not as Hegel said, "The owl of Minerva flies only in the dusk," or people only wake up too late.

May 25, 2022

Have we dodged the bullet? Geert, one of the heroes of this virus disaster, may be wrong, at least temporarily. This gets kinda complicated, but I will try not to oversimplify.

His concern was that the needle would stimulate the neutralizing antibodies at the expense of the non-neutralizing, which protects the lower respiratory tract. The Wuhan virus, by now, has escaped the neutralizing antibodies. If it escapes the non-neutralizing antibodies, then it affects the lower respiratory tract and becomes more virulent, much more lethal, and then we have a perfect storm.

So far, this hasn't happened. But the Wuhan virus will not go away until the non-needled population with naturally acquired immunity gets big enough. If they needle the kids, then there will be no reservoir of immunity in the Western world, and the only hope for humanity would be the non-needled from Africa and Asia. We all hope Geert is wrong, but so far, he has been right every time.

I have just been listening to Reiner Fuellmich, the lawyer who is attempting to oversee the International Criminal Court, set up in July 2021. I have intermittently listened to the evidence provided by various doctors, vaccinologists, and scientists regarding the disastrous handling of this very questionable PCR test and the subsequent lockdown.

Psychologists have testified to the induction of what they call "mass formation psychosis," a process whereby most of the population becomes mentally ill, for example, in Germany in the '30s. Most of the world, in 2020 and 2021, appears to have undergone a similar phenomenon, allowing themselves to be locked up for a year or more for a tightly targeted virus, which had essentially no effect on most of the population. And then rushing to accept an experimental gene therapy needle with no long-term data.

This mass-formation psychosis seems to be waning, but it is still there and may be reactivated by the fear porn being produced by the legacy media about a few cases of monkeypox.

Fuellmich is deeply concerned that this conflict in Eastern Europe will spill over and engulf the world. Surely not! But listening to the increasing drumbeat of fear and misinformation, who knows what will happen. Deus Vult. Surely, sanity will return.

Comment

1. For two years now the MSM has presented a daily deluge of fear porn and virus misinformation. The fear of interaction with others is still there, even inside families. The legacy media and WHO seem determined to keep this going. Are we smart enough to resist?

A. Seeing a fair number of people walking around outside on their own, wearing these silly face masks, one despairs. Under such circumstances, the face mask is the diagnostic symbol of the psychosis, which is likely permanently embedded in their brain.

June 2, 2022

Lots of kids are in the medical clinic today, many with lockdown disease. Sore legs, backs, and feet from unaccustomed activity. After two years in jail, they are out of shape, obese, weak, and afraid. It makes you want to weep.

Thinking of Rupert Brooke, the WWI poet who died in that futile, meaningless war. These young heroes thought they were dying for something. Everyone in my generation knows his lines,

> If I should die, think only this of me:
> That there's some corner of a foreign field
> That is forever England.

But what I am really thinking of is his other poem:

> These laid the world away
> Poured out the red sweet wine of youth
> Gave up the years to be of work and joy.

That's what the last two years have done.

Fortunately, this unnecessary war in Europe is far away, and hopefully, my kids will never be involved. But it is not just war; it is the detritus of two years of lockdown. And just when you think the madness is going away, although in Canada we still have silly, meaningless restrictions, lo and behold, the money pox—sorry, monkeypox—has just arrived. Rumor has it, it is from the same place, and the same players are involved.

Already one hears the drumbeat of quarantine, AKA lockdown, and another mandatory needle. And masks. Chaps, masking was a joke and a hoax for an airborne virus, and this money pox is a disease of prolonged physical contact, really an STD.

We have eventually discovered why there is a shortage of baby formula in the US. I hear that the FDA closed the plant because they thought there was a problem. Turns out there was none, but they forgot to authorize reopening. They also block the importation of baby food from Europe. Is this deliberate or simply another example of bureaucratic incompetence?

Anyway, the sun is shining and my backyard tomato plants are growing. They cost so much this year that there will have to be runaway inflation before I break even.

June 9, 2022

SADS, sudden adult death syndrome! Have you heard of it? I am sure that you have seen it with young, fit professional soccer and other athletes dropping dead on the field. And no one knows the cause! Doctors claim to be puzzled by the acute onset of this new condition. What is new in the last eighteen months to explain it? Perhaps global warming.

Those puzzled doctors make you think of the ditty,

See the happy moron,
He doesn't give a damn,
I wish I were a moron,
My God! perhaps I am.

One thing which has changed in the last eighteen months is that vast numbers have been needled and boosted, except Africa, especially Tanzania, which rejected the fake PCR test after a goat and breadfruit tested positive. They also rejected the needle. Increasingly, it looks like Africa was right and the rest of the world was wrong. It was the African delegates who recently halted the attempted takeover by WHO. They seem to have saved us from "*La Trahison des Clercs*," as Benda wrote ("The treachery of the intellectuals.)

The insurance company actuaries and dry, bloodless mathematicians point to the unexpected rise in deaths in the preretirement age group for no clear reason. And some heroic US army docs have documented the catastrophic rise in deaths and disease in the young, fit military people. And yet we are not allowed to speculate about the cause. As Confucius said in 500 BC, "An oppressive government is more to be feared than a tiger."

Similarly, there is rising hysteria about money pox—sorry, monkeypox. There are several issues. Firstly, it is really only spread by very intimate contact, such as sex. Mandatory masking as suggested by the ever-trustworthy, ever-truthful CDC makes no sense. Secondly, I hear that a version of the PCR test is being used for diagnosis. Given its 97 percent inaccurate track record, it is hardly diagnostic. I also hear via the grapevine that many of the money pox cases are, in fact, herpes or shingles reactivated by repeated boosters. I am sure that is just a rumor along with the one that both originated in the same lab funded by the same sainted doctor.

Truth is hard to find nowadays. But if reduced immunity is going to lead to disaster, then rather than end in a war that the war hawks keep pushing for, the needle may prove to be the great extinction. Maybe T. S. Eliot is right.

> *This is the way the world ends*
> *This is the way the world ends*
> *Not with a bang but a whimper.*
>
> —"The Hollow Men"

If so, before we go, I hope we wake up and listen to Hosea, that "those who have sown the wind shall reap the whirlwind."

But surely not! Surely, this is just a bad dream, and we will all awaken tomorrow, and everything will be as it was before the fall of 2019.

Comments

1. The only thing which has changed is the needle. I commented on that, but FB hid my comment.
2. Who decides which comment is relevant? It appears the doctor's comment has been hidden. The realization that everything we thought was real is actually not, is daunting. I wish this was simply a dream.
3. You are right. Truth is hard to find.

June 20, 2022

To paraphrase Francis Thompson:

> We fled them down the nights and down the days,
> We fled them, down the arches of the years."

We are fleeing the edicts of the sainted Dr. F, WHO, the CDC, and others who pursue us with needles and mandates.

The excess mortality data from most countries shows that if we had never heard of the virus from you-know-where, we would never have noticed. It was not, after all, the relatively harmless virus that produced such devastation. It was the incredible, manufactured overreaction to it. Stupidity can't be used as an excuse. Even a moron is right occasionally, but the decisions and edicts of the sainted Dr. F, the public health Johnnies, and the CDC have been 100 percent wrong.

Dr. Shetty, one of the many ignored docs who got it right, talks about the "snobbery of the experts." But these people, Dr. F and the public health Johnnies, were bureaucrats, not experts. And when did anyone ever expect a bureaucrat to be right about anything? They are examples of Fermat's last theorem: Do worthless people become bureaucrats or does becoming a bureaucrat make people worthless?

The main driver worldwide of this tragedy was the PCR test. As most people now know, Kary Mullis, who got the Nobel Prize for developing this technology, said that it was never to be used in this way. Run at a multiplier of 42, as it was in Canada and many other countries, it was worthless, as up to 97 percent were false positives. It produced the only epidemic in history where you had to take a test to know you had a disease when you were not ill.

Lockdown and all the other Faucian measures, such as masking and distancing, were totally contrary to all Western medicine and even the WHO rules until they were changed in 2020. They have been responsible for the starving kids in the Third World and the damaged kids in the developed world who will pay for this lunacy for the rest of their lives?

And the needle! Docs are still afraid to talk about it, as they may lose their license. I have heard it described as the Tuskegee experiment on kids, as there is no long-term data. All we can say, because it is public knowledge, is that it doesn't stop infection or transmission and the data from Israel suggests no effect on mortality. So why is it still being pushed? Is this the depopulation sought by some?

To paraphrase T S Elliot, is this the way the world ends, not with a bang but a whimper?

Comments

1. It is beginning to feel that we are beset by those who are determined to destroy everything that makes up civil society.
2. Yep. The fallout continues.
3. I finally caught it after two years. I was sick for a while, just like the flu. But I am OK now.

June 26, 2022

"What news from the Rialto, Antonio?" asks the Merchant of Venice. That was when Rialto was, in some sense, the economic center of Europe. Well, something surprising! I just heard on YouTube a couple of clever scientists talking about the virus from you know where. I still worry about being deplatformed if one states the obvious. They were puzzled by the behavior of the virus. If clever people with no financial interest are puzzled, then sit up and listen.

In my own field of orthopedic surgery, I would occasionally hear interesting things late at night in dim bars in Korea or Frankfurt or other places. If two smart doctors from different parts of the world were telling me that something was wrong, but they didn't know what exactly, I always listened, as I wrote in my book, *Have Knife Will Travel.* I usually acted on these whispers in the wind. By doing so, I saved myself and my patients a world of hurt.

So what are these new whispers? They think that Omicron, Delta, and the original virus do not have much linear relationship. We knew that the insertion of the original furin cleavage site had no connections to a natural virus. But the suggestion that Omicron and Delta do not have much of a relationship is new.

They wondered how many viruses were in those leaky fridges in Wuhan, as it might need different culture techniques to produce such dissimilar viruses. One speculated that Omicron was actually a new living transmittable vaccine, which had been released by someone feeling guilty about the disaster of the original virus and the resulting mandatory needles. Omicron, after all, acts like a vaccine. That sounds really tin hat, but then, it does make some sense.

The current needle neither stops infection nor transmission or as seems to be the case in Israel, hospitalization. The other effects are unknown but seem endless and are not good.

And what else is going on? Hysteria is being whipped up about the money pox—sorry, monkeypox. Research on this was apparently being done in the same lab, funded by the same people. The date of release, amazingly, was accurately predicted about a year ago. And now there is hysteria about polio. In Europe, they are talking about masking again, in spite of knowing that all that ever did was damage kids.

It is all so strange. Maybe my new books, *Betrayal* and *Rogue Pharma*, are not fiction. With all these young men dropping dead, the Four Horsemen of the Apocalypse, war, famine, plague, and Death seem to be riding through the world. Is this a non-kinetic version of Ragnarök, the battle at the end of time?

Comment

1. We live in strange and dangerous times.

A. Who knows what. Is Omicron actually a proper vaccine? All we know is that if it is reported by the legacy media. Believe the opposite.

July 4, 2022

The sky is falling! The plague has returned! Soon universal masking will be mandatory in New Zealand, Australia, and possibly Canada. We are not sure why, but the legacy media is sounding the trumpets.

It is one of life's mysteries why these mask fanatics don't speak to someone who knows about masking, like a spray painter or drywaller. They will explain particle size and how universal masking is a hoax and a joke. We surgeons use masks in the operating room to avoid blood splashes and drooling into the wound. There is, however, almost no evidence that masking reduces wound infection.

If you actually want to reduce infection from an airborne virus, a respirator would be necessary, as in a level-4 lab. They can be used for a short time only as they are uncomfortable. Users have to be trained on how to put them on and take them off. And how do you re-sterilize them? So thousands knew that universal masking made no sense.

We did know or were pretty certain of the damage universal masking would do to kids who were never at any risk from the virus. The delayed development and education were predictable. Kids in Europe were never masked. None of this was rocket science.

What is so inexplicable is that, in spite of the fact that thousands knew this was futile, the politicians and the public health Johnnies pushed ahead with it. Did they actually believe what they were trumpeting? Possibly, given the incredible damage done to the energy sector and world economy by the global warmists who clearly don't know much about anything. Was this disaster planned? Surely not.

And now the money pox—sorry, monkeypox. Surely, not from the same lab funded by the same players.

Ah well, it is summer in Canada. So as it says in the *Rubáiyát*,

> Make the most of what we yet may spend,
> Before we too into the Dust descend.

So get outside and soak up some vitamin D while it lasts. As Shakespeare wrote that 'summer's lease has all too short a course.'

Comment

1. It seems that the emphasis is on distraction while our WEF clone leaders continue to destroy our economies and freedoms.

A. A reasonable conclusion to draw, under the circumstances.

July 8, 2022

Sitting in the medical clinic today, doing nothing as our internet provider crashed hours ago. The parking lot is full of hot and bothered and angry patients waiting! Waiting for permission to enter, which we can only give via the internet.

Waiting is the symbol of our times. Everywhere we go, waiting. Airports are a disaster as a result of silly government rules; sea ports and supply chains are in disarray; hospitals, energy, fuel, and farming are a disaster. How did this happen?

Listen to Mattias Desmet, the famed Belgian psychologist, explain it. He says Hannah Arendt described it in her 1963 book, *The Banality of Evil.* This is a new form of totalitarianism. It is the rise of the "expert." But these people, like the sainted Dr. F, are not experts. They are bureaucrats. At one time, they may have known something, but that was a long time ago.

The way up the control ladder in organizations like the CDC, or the civil service, is not through expertise. It is the ability to tolerate endless meetings, meetings upon meetings, committees upon committees, all day every day for years. These are the people who are promoted and end up running things. They are the Adolph Eichmann's of this world.

The goal of a bureaucrat is a promotion to run a bigger department and have a bigger pension. Everything else is secondary. What happens to the populace as a result of their disastrous recommendations is of no concern. When did you ever hear of a bureaucrat being fired for incompetence? It doesn't happen.

The response to this none-too-serious virus exemplifies that. All traditional Western medicine was discarded with what are now obviously tragic results. Similarly, this global warming farce has led to energy shortages and coming mass starvation. The rule of the bureaucratic experts is responsible for this. Politicians are mostly lawyers who know nothing, and so, depend on bureaucrats whom they regard as experts.

So what is the answer? One feels like Augustine, the bishop of Hippo, watching the lights going out in Rome. "It is finished," he said, and it was for one thousand years.

But surely not! Who will stand against the twin terrors of the bureaucrats and Davos! Somewhere out there is Martin Luther, William Tell, or Jan Sobieski. Deus Vult!

Comments

1. The one-world, uber-authoritarian cabal can destroy with great efficiency. If they fulfill their promise to "Build Back Better," it will be the first time totalitarians have succeeded in improving any society they extinguish.
2. This does seem much like the end of this phase of civilization.
3. Fini!

A. How unutterably sad. As Kipling wrote,

> Low among the alders lie the derelict foundations,
> The beams whereon they trusted and the plinths whereon
> they built—
>
> - "The Song of Seven Cities"

July 12, 2022

I am at a medical clinic this morning in the least wealthy area in Toronto. So many people are admirable, struggling in the midst of terrible adversity.

All around us, we see the Western world; indeed, looking at Sri Lanka, the whole world collapsing. The four horsemen of the Apocalypse are riding out: war, famine, plague, and Death. And yet these disadvantaged patients struggle with few complaints. It is an honor to serve them.

The global warmists are at it again, trying to stop farming in Holland, the UK, and the US. The problem in Sri Lanka is the government banned fertilizer, so the rice crop collapsed. Is this due to incompetence or is it deliberate? Nothing but bugs and algae to eat, and you only get to eat if you obey.

Australia and NZ, once the poster boys of lockdown, still have not realized that you can't keep out a highly infectious, low-morbidity, airborne virus. They claim their health care system is near collapse with flu cases. This is the Hygiene Hypothesis created by the lockdown come true and, possibly, additional loss of immunity due to repeated needles. And yet they want more needles and a return to the futile masking. I guess they have never heard of the Johns Hopkins report, which confirmed what everyone knew, that mandates were less than worthless, and of Israel, whose data has shown boosters of no significant help.

Is this chaos what the Great Reset is all about? *Dies irae, dies illa*! The day of wrath, that dreadful day when heaven and earth shall pass away.

July 17, 2022

The Pandemic Industrial Complex! I just heard that term. It explains exactly what has been happening for the last two years.

Eisenhower tried to warn the world about the Military-Industrial Complex. Think of how many pointless, unnecessary wars have been waged since then. The explanations of why the West should repeatedly go to war get less and less believable.

Mea culpa! I was so naïve. Until the last two years, I sort of believed a little of what the legacy media reported. Now I believe exactly the opposite. Bismarck, the Iron Chancellor, was right as usual when he said "nothing should be believed until it has been officially denied." If only he had still been running Germany, I am sure that the bloodbath of WWI would never have occurred. I am now so distrustful that I actually wonder if the City of London was not at the bottom of that disaster.

I even wonder about the Twin Towers, as their collapse never made engineering sense. Was that just another Gulf of Tonkin or weapons of mass destruction? Who knows! The fact I now question these events surprises even me.

Even if the NIH-funded virus accidentally escaped in May 2019, the subsequent events do fit with the Pandemic Industrial Complex. Ask yourself, Cui bono? Cherchez la femme; follow the money?

If that's true, the incredible viciousness of big tech and the legacy media in closing down the debate makes sense. No questions at all were allowed. And look who funds the formerly trustworthy agencies like the FDA, the CDC, and the NIH. Who made money out of the lockdown, and who continues to make money from this ridiculous random virus testing of visitors to Canada? Who will make money if the farmers are not allowed to farm? Who is producing fake food?

So where will this end? The leaders of the valiant Canadian truckers are still in jail. Is this what the Dutch, Italian, Spanish, and German farmers are facing? Or is the sleeping giant finally waking? As Chesterton wrote,

> The last lingering troubadour to whom the bird has sung [of freedom],
> That once went singing southward when all the world was young.
> In that enormous silence, tiny and unafraid,
> Comes up along a winding road the noise of the [farmers] Crusade.
>
> —"Lepanto"

Comments

1. Welcome to reality. Of course the Twin Towers were a false flag event. I have been trying to sound the alarm since the Gulf of Tonkin incident in 1964.
2. For some time now some very bad actors have been saying that population reduction is the goal.

A. It is scary when you think about who is in authority and who can make decisions.

July 24, 2022

Are the tractors of the Dutch farmers the "chariots of fire?" Looking around at the tragedy of the last few years and the monsters coming unashamedly out of the closet, I had begun to think that all was lost, that "the days of wine and roses" were finished.

I was drawn unwillingly into this sewer by the NIH-funded virus. Not the virus, which wasn't much of a predator, but the unbelievable reaction to it. By May 2020, we knew something was wrong, really, really wrong. I then began to hear whispers that something had been strange about the AIDS epidemic and, in particular, H1N1. In retrospect, was that a dress rehearsal for the Wuhan virus or a failed attempt? It featured the same people. Google "Jane Burgermeister," the woman who blew the whistle on that one, and what they did to her in revenge.

Joseph Schumpeter said that in a decent society, the workers would produce enough money to fund a useless drone or chattering class who produce nothing and hate the workers. Obviously, this has happened. Universities and HR departments are full of poorly educated, semi-literate people who do not understand that they have been indoctrinated by the Frankfurt school. Their sole goal in life is to spread this indoctrination to naïve and slightly dull four-year liberal arts degree students. You see the product of this nightly on the legacy media.

I have come to believe that we, the people, face the triple threat of the military-industrial complex, the Frankfurt school, and fresh out of the closet, the WEF. But to that, we must now add the plandemic industrial complex. They were openly discussing the release of a coronavirus before it happened, and a year ago gave the date of release of monkeypox.

It looks like the West is doomed. But there is a Japanese word, *ikigai*, which means "a reason for being," that you are alive for a purpose. The first of those who got off their knees and stood up to this monstrous tyranny was the Canadian truckers. Justine, the acolyte of Klaus of Davos, showed how far these oligarchs of the new world order were prepared to go, crushing them by declaring martial law and freezing their bank accounts. Undeterred, the people of Sri Lanka and the Dutch farmers have risen up. It looks like the other European farmers are also on the march.

Is the Reconquista? Have the people finally gotten off their knees to oppose those who would enslave them? Deus Vult!

Comment

1. Let us have hope that ordinary people will rise against this tyranny.

July 31, 2022

It can't be true! It must be a nightmare! The dear leader of Canada is joining the WEF leaders in Sri Lanka and Holland in stopping farmers from using fertilizer.

As a simple surgeon, I never thought I would be writing about politics, but the obvious falseness of the response to the NIH-funded none-too-serious virus forced reality on many of us to see the world as it really is, not as one would like it to be.

It seems so sad that all the triumphs and glories of the West are being destroyed in front of our eyes by a James Bond comic book villain. Hiding in his mountain lair, he sends out his uncaring, handsome, utterly incompetent underlings like Justine, Jacinda, Rutte, and others to destroy the world as we know it. We watch with horror the lights going out in Europe, even before the beginning of winter. Hot water is already rationed. With the burning of food processing plants and the banning of fertilizer, great hunger is coming.

Maybe it is simply due to incompetence, but Klaus has openly boasted about reducing the number of "worthless eaters," as he calls ordinary people. We thought, when the wall came down, that the horror of socialist collectivism had gone. We should have listened to the Russian defector, Yuri Bezmenov. Sadly, it has come to pass exactly as he laid it out. If you want to have nightmares, google him.

Just before the release of the virus in 2019, the world seemed so good with lots of cheap and reliable energy and abundant food. It collapsed so rapidly that the termites were obviously in the building foundations. One of the bureaucrats, in large part responsible for the disastrous lockdown, has just admitted that she was knowingly lying. And incredibly, no one cares! That's what we expect from bureaucrats.

I can't believe what I have just written. It sounds crazy, end-of-the-world stuff, really tin hat. I must be wrong. It must be a nightmare after all, and I will wake up soon. Won't I?

Comments

1. No fertilizer, no farmers, no food, no future. I am afraid you have once again nailed it.
2. We must continue to fight the false narrative these evil elites are promulgating.

A. We pray for the farmers to succeed, but the legacy media refuse to cover the protests so the future looks bleak.

August 3, 2022

Another good man down! A TGH nurse we have known for fifty years has just called to commiserate about the passing of an orthopedic surgeon and friend, John Cameron.

A life well lived. John was responsible for defining a knee problem that bedeviled young women. John Cameron and his discoveries are featured in the book Edna Quammie and I wrote about Toronto General Hospital, *The Big House (1972 to 1984).* That alone would justify his life. But he was much more, a colleague, a friend, and a man of honor.

Ave atque vale, John Cameron.

Comment

That epitaph got responses from all over the world. Hundreds mourned the loss of a good man,

August 7, 2022

"This is crazy!" I was thinking this when I selected a much-used paper face mask from the pile on the back seat of my car. I put it on to go into the clinic to start my shift. In Canada, we are forced to use these useless, soiled masks in medical clinics and hospitals. I kid you not! In Canada, in August 2022.

Surely, by now, even the dullest public health Johnny, and many are clearly really, really intellectually challenged, should know that there is not a shred of credible evidence that these soiled, reused masks are of any value. The CDC and the sainted Dr. F still claim they should be used, but who believes these fallen icons?

There is ample credible evidence of the harm masking has done to children intellectually and, almost certainly, psychologically. And yet, some states are planning on re-masking kids. Don't they know it was never done to little kids in Europe?

I guess also they have never heard of the Hygiene Hypothesis. If little kids are not exposed to a wide range of bugs and viruses, their immune systems don't develop properly. The large outbreaks of a dangerous childhood condition called Respiratory Syncytial Virus in New Zealand and Australia are thought to be the result of the prolonged lockdown. Others, such as childhood hepatitis, seem to be on the way.

Initially, I thought that the ludicrous response to the virus was a combination of stupidity, fear, and in the case of WHO, corruption. By 2021, it was obvious that greed also played a major role. Like everyone else, I found it difficult to believe the cartoon James Bond villain squatting on his mountaintop in Davos was real.

But the banning of fertilizer is real, as seen by the starvation in Sri

Lanka, a country that used to export food. And now fertilizer is being banned by the Klaus groupies in Holland, Canada, Ireland, and other places. If they succeed, then in addition to freezing in the dark because cheap and reliable energy has been banned, we will also starve.

The oncoming disaster will make the Great Leap Forward of Mao when thirty million Chinese starved to death, look like a trivial accident.

This surely can't be true, can it?

Comment

1. All are carefully documented in our wonderful legacy media. Not a single word. They are bought and sold.

A. In Canada, the federal government funds the legacy media so there is, of course, never any criticism.

August 18, 2022

Another day, another gentle, despairing rant! The sun is shining, and the downtown hospital office is quiet, so maybe go outside for a walk. But a senior-floor nurse just dropped by to say hello. She is as fit, vigorous, and smart as the day I met her thirty years ago. She is so fed up with the useless hospital rules, she is thinking of walking away and quitting. What a tragedy!

Outside the US, the health care systems in the Anglo world are collapsing. I don't know about other countries, but I just had a patient from Portugal, and he said it is just as bad there. I had a three-year-old in my clinic the other day. She needs a five-minute operation. The children's hospital says they are only seeing emergencies. Private practice is banned in Canada. So what should the mom do? Go to India?

The CDC just admitted that the needle doesn't do much. If you compare Gaza and Israel, you have known that for months. So why can't the nurses and others, who knew it was unnecessary and refused it, get their jobs back? Are they being punished for being sensible?

I worked on farms as a boy, but everyone who grows tomatoes in their backyard knows you fertilize them. So why are the "young leaders" of Klaus of Davos, who seem to run most Western countries, banning fertilizer? Don't they know what happened in Sri Lanka? That island went from a food exporter to hunger. Is worldwide starvation really their goal? We know they want to sell fake food and bugs, but is starvation necessary? That sounds so silly, but what other explanation is there? Stupidity, while it may be true, is hardly an adequate explanation.

The good news is Denmark has banned the needle for kids. But when will the rest of the world wake up?

Hegel wrote that the owl of Minerva flies only in the dusk. Meaning people only wake up when it is too late. I hope not! I really hope not!

Comment

1. The origin of the virus was always suspicious, as so many influential people were making so much money out of it. My friends thought I was wrong to avoid the needle, but now many have told me, "No more boosters."

A. It is hard to blame normal people who knew nothing about medicine and were subjected to this constant drumbeat of fear, and this insistence that the needle was salvation.

August 28, 2022

It's morning and the sun is shining. Thinking Pippa's song:

> God's in His heaven—
> All's right with the world."

And then you listen to YouTube, disaster all around. You think of Marcel Proust, echoing Boethius, "The true paradises are the paradises that we have lost."

Where did the looming disaster of starvation and no energy come from? Three years ago, everything was great—no wars, no famine, no plague, and cheap energy. Then suddenly, the Four Horsemen of the Apocalypse appear—war, famine, plague, and death. All manmade! How did we get here?

The institutions were obviously becoming corrupt—the UN, WHO, the CDC, the deep state, the legacy media, and sadly, the universities. The rise of the laptop class, the administrators! Parkinson's law states that administration increases by 4 percent per year. That is certainly an underestimate. In keeping with the Pareto principle at least 80 percent of these people have essentially nothing to do, so they pass new rules and regulations and multiply. The more staff they have, obviously, the more important they are, and the more they need to be paid. Look at any medical system.

Then there is funding. Increased government funding means increased control; dissent is verboten, as in the Canadian legacy media. University professors need funding for research, essential for promotion, so they produce the results the funder wants. Look at the corruption of global warming as exposed by Climategate, and no one cared. Couple this with the Long March of the Frankfurt school, with socialism taking over education, the media, entertainment, and politics.

We were like lemmings looking over the edge of the abyss, and we didn't know. All it took was the release of a none-too-serious virus, and the whole edifice of civilization collapsed.

The population accepted jail, called lockdown. The middle class was bankrupted. With more than one hundred million (UN estimates) looking at starvation with unbelievably no serious protests, the elites have now banned fertilizer. No fertilizer, no food. Dutch farmers are protesting, but the government and media are ignoring it. Other countries, including Canada, are also banning fertilizer.

But why? What is the end game of those who must know that their policies will produce mass starvation? Is it to sell fake food? Is the goal depopulation as many have stated? Is it really simply a desire to return to the days of millions of starving serfs and a few overlords? What do you think?

Comments

1. You can add the media to the list of the corrupt.
2. The boiling frog! The screaming won't begin until it is too late. We tried to appeal with facts and reason. Why didn't you tell us they will cry? I'll smile and be glad I am old.
3. At least we had fun in the seventies.

A. If you assume the voting isn't rigged, which it very well might be, then one has to assume that those who vote for the Klaus of Davos clones are indeed the frogs in the pot. And yes, we certainly did have fun in the seventies. What a wonderful time—whiskey; cigarettes; and wild, wild women.

September 4, 2022

I was grocery shopping and, on instinct, bought reams of toilet paper. You know what that means. Toilet paper shortage is the best indicator of a looming economic disaster. *Dies irae, dies illa* (The day of wrath that dreadful day.) I hear some paper mills in Germany have closed, as they can't afford the energy to keep them open.

When the Berlin Wall came down in 1989, we thought we were looking at peace and prosperity forever. But in 2022, Europe and much of the world are looking at starvation in the cold and dark. It is beginning to resemble 1816, the year of no summer, due to the volcanic eruption of Mt. Tambora. That starvation was due to a natural disaster, but this one is manmade due to the deliberate action of a small group of people.

A couple of years ago I would have thought such a statement was crazy, lunacy, tin hat stuff. But then the Plandemic or Scamdemic, whatever you like to call it, happened, exactly as outlined in Event 201 in October 2019. Initially, we were fooled by the misinformation from WHO and others. By May 2020, we knew something was wrong.

Left alone, a highly infectious, low-morbidity, airborne virus would blow through the population in a month or two after it triggered. Lockdown, if it had any effect at all, and then the needle, encouraged mutation exactly as Geert and Knut predicted.

For years, the global warmists had been deliberately destroying the basis of modern civilization—cheap and reliable energy. The results of these policies, coupled with the supply chain disruption caused by the lockdown, resulted in a perfect storm. And now the followers of Klaus of Davos are banning fertilizer to add starvation to the mix. The protests of the farmers, who actually grow the food are being ignored. So, shortly, we will be looking at the same disaster as Sri Lanka, which went from a food exporter to starvation.

I heard it said that if we stare into the abyss for long enough, we will see light. I hope so. I really hope so.

Comment

1. Don't worry! Bill has the situation under control. You can order your crickets medium rare, delivered by drone.

A. Fake food for all you peasants, eh?

September 8, 2022

At the hospital this morning. I have been on staff there since 1982. I went around some of the wards. Where are all the senior nurses I knew? A superb ward clerk I have known for decades has had enough; she told me she is taking a package and walking away.

I had an OR nurse from a first-class general hospital in my clinic the other day. She says a quarter of the ORs in her hospital are closed due to a lack of nurses. My hospital is an elective orthopedic hospital with no sick patients. This morning, there were masses of young girls the government is trying to rush through nursing to make up for the missing experienced nurses who walked away when threatened with the needle. I am sure these young people will be fine in time.

At least, a tiny flicker of sanity. A Canadian university, which, at the last moment, after the kids had paid for the tuition, mandated the needle, has backed down due to the storm of protests. Even the CDC admits that the needle isn't of much value, and the data about the side effects gets worse almost daily. So why did that university insist?

In Canada, the dear leader is again threatening to mandate the needle for everyone. Unbelievable! The new data from Israel on the cover-up of the side effects of the needle is simply shocking, and surely, heads will roll after such an admission of culpability and damage. "Following orders" was not accepted as an excuse at Nuremberg.

If the fertility data from Europe is correct, there will be a lot fewer of us in the next few decades. Eighteen months ago, even the totally discredited WHO estimated that millions would starve as a result of the lockdown and supply chain disruption. If the followers of Klaus of Davos get their way and fertilizer is banned, there will be a lot fewer of us a lot sooner than you think.

Why are they doing this? Is this Agenda 21? Is this what it is all about? What do you think?

Comments

1. Depopulation is their stated goal. What is so foolish is that Elon Musk has pointed out that in a few decades, lack of population will be the problem as it already is in Japan, Korea, and other places.
2. I have read Ontario alone has lost over ten young doctors to Sudden Adult Death Syndrome.

A. The number of dead young doctors is closer to twenty and growing. The authorities say it is a mystery and want to needle kids. As far as population goes, once a culture becomes wealthy enough, especially when women are educated, population growth declines precipitously. So if it is felt there are too many people, then educate the women and increase the GNP of the poor of the world.

September 16, 2022

Have you heard of the Hygiene Hypothesis? Lots of little sick kids. In Ontario, Canada, they have been locked up for years with silly police tape around kids' amusements and compulsory masking. Their immunity is weak, as they have not been exposed to the numerous viruses floating around. So when they finally go back to school, they get sick with a virus they normally would not notice.

In New Zealand and Australia, there have been lots of kids sick with Respiratory Syncytial Virus. Even hepatitis is occurring, possibly due to a normally mild adenovirus. Who knows!

Lockdown, social distancing, and masking were contrary to all Western medicine. We knew by May 2020 it was silly, ineffectual, and wickedly destructive. The collateral deaths from this failed policy are already likely far higher than from the none-too-serious, age-stratified virus. In Africa, with no PCR test and no needle, there have been few deaths. But there will be from a supply chain collapse due to the lockdown.

Not content with this disastrous nonscientific policy, we are facing the consequences of this failed green energy doctrine, and we now have a war with sanctions causing further havoc in the West. At this moment, with the world teetering on the edge of disaster, the Davos crowd is banning fertilizer. They succeeded in changing Sri Lanka from a food exporter to starvation. And yet in Canada, Holland, Ireland, and many other countries, the same policies are being enacted.

None of this makes sense unless worldwide collapse is their goal. That sounds ridiculous, but what do you think?

Comment

1. Ottawa's disastrous edicts and mandates and deliberately inflationary policies in lockstep with Davos are creating a desperate time for Canadians.

A. The economic world ranking of Canada continues on a downward trajectory. Every federal government failure and every economic misstep is airily passed off as a "good thing" to "save the planet."

September 26, 2022

Good news! perhaps. I hear our dear leader in Canada is lifting travel restrictions. But what does this mean? I hear that random testing of travelers will still be enforced. Unbelievable! Random testing tells one nothing about anything. Just another irritant and invasion of privacy. It is exactly the same as the other silly mandates, scientifically meaningless but financially rewarding to some. Perhaps that is the reason.

By May 2020 we knew that this virus was tightly targeted at the ill elderly, the morbidly obese, and severely diabetics. Even in these groups, the death rate was a little higher than in a bad flu year.

So where was this epidemic? Kary Mullis, who got the Nobel for developing the PCR technique, said it was never to be used in this way, as run at a high enough CT, it could be made to show anything. Possibly run at 20, a few million times multiplier, it might mean something. In Canada, it was run at 42, a few trillion times multiplier and produced what was thought to be 97 percent false positives. These false positives were called 'cases' where no one was sick. This was therefore a Casedemic (i.e., something with no meaning), not an epidemic.

In Africa where the PCR test and needle were ignored, and there was no epidemic.

With the exception of the CDC, university administrators, and the public health Johnnies everyone knows that the needle doesn't stop infection or transmission. The data from Israel suggests, if anything, the needle makes one more liable to infection. So why force it on those who don't need it?

Starvation is coming with the banning of fertilizer and freezing with the banning of energy. Is another lockdown coming to prevent the free people from taking to the streets?

I just heard the good news from Europe about the Italian federal election, or we hope it is good news. Viva Italia. Perhaps a little sanity returning. Only time will tell.

Comment

1. A friend said her daughter coming through the airport was picked for a random test which she had to pay for herself!

A. I suppose some friend of a friend in authority is making money from it. I can't think of any other reason. There certainly is no medical one.

October 7, 2022

I have no idea what is happening. FB keeps changing things. I don't know if anyone can see this or if I have finally been shadow-banned completely. If I have, then I guess that's that. It was nice knowing you. Ave atque vale, hail and farewell. If the West finally defeats Klaus of Davos and his sycophants then we will meet again.

Shadow-banning. I got eighty-one comments saying that they had not been seeing my posts for a long time. So I guess shadow-banning is real. Somehow, in the confusion at FB, this post sneaked through the filter. I suspected it. I suppose there is nothing that can be done about it.

October 10, 2022

Thank you all for your support in the last couple of days. I thought all was lost to the fury of the fact-checkers.

"What is truth?" said Pontius Pilate, faced with a kangaroo court, lying witnesses, and corrupt and incompetent bureaucrats. I always thought he sounded utterly weary; a good man trapped in an impossible situation. Just like Jeffery Sachs (google him).

Sachs was appointed to head up the US inquiry into the origin of the virus. As an economist, he knew nothing about science. It took him a long time to realize that every "expert" on his committee was evading the truth. He eventually realized that they were all controlled by the sainted Dr. F, who controlled the funding from the NIH. In science, if there is no funding, then there is no research, so no promotion and no future. So in the US, all medical scientists and doctors dance to the Faucian tune. I am sure it is the same in all Western countries.

Reviewing my posts from the spring of 2020, it was obvious, even to me, a simple orthopedic surgeon with an obsolete iPhone, that information showed that the virus was created in 2018 or earlier. The fear was that HIV, stolen from the lab in Winnipeg, had been added, which would mean no immunity ever. But then, acting under orders from the sainted Dr. F, social media began censorship.

I knew the PCR test was fake as did thousands of others. Videos of Kary Mullis, who developed the technology, are still available, saying it was never to be used like this. I recently found that they had tried to do the same thing with H1N1, but Jane Burgermeister (google her) blew the whistle.

This time, as they had almost complete control of the legacy media, they got away with it, locking down the world for the bad flu and forcing gene therapy, relabeled as a "needle," onto millions of people. Fortunately, some honest governments have woken up and are banning it for young people. After this tragedy, many people, especially parents, will never trust a needle again, even the time-tested good ones.

With the Davos crowd trying to ban fertilizer to create starvation, ban energy, and start WWIII, sitting in my office, all I could see ahead was doom and gloom. But then, a very, very senior Persian lady patient who, for family reasons, is just learning how to cook, brought me homemade lunch. And then a senior-covered lady brought me a big basket of spinach and green peppers from her own garden. So it could be worse. Google Peter Brueghel's *The Peasant Wedding*, 1567. While we live, there is hope.

Comments

1. I am totally tired of these experts in health, global warming, finance, and any other money-making field. Many, if not most, are funded by someone who will profit from their "advice" to the unsuspecting public.
2. I looked up the Brueghel painting. Thanks for the little extra gift. I learned of a new artist today.

A. They had some good times even in the Dark Ages. The Dutch masters have always been my favorite artists, especially the Van Ruisdael landscapes. And "experts," most you see in the media are, in fact, bureaucrats, has-beens, or never-weres.

October 19, 2022

What is this madness? Were the end-of-time guys in the tin hats correct? I always thought that the revelations of St. John the Divine were a magic-mushroom-induced nightmarish vision. But look at what is happening.

WAR – we have a war produced deliberately by ignoring the Treaty of Minsk and the expansion eastward of NATO. Why? Who does it benefit other than the military-industrial complex?

PLAGUE—we know the virus was produced by the insertion of the furin cleavage site developed in NC and taught to the Bat Woman. The US funding for more of the same gain-of-function research in Wuhan continues. Boston has just produced an infinitely worse virus. Why?

FAMINE—this is being produced by the banning of fertilizer in multiple countries. Sri Lanka went from a food exporter to starvation, and yet, they are banning it in Holland, many European countries, Canada, etc. Why?

DEATH—more than forty young Canadian docs have unexpectedly died this year. Excess deaths are spiking all over the needled world. Some countries have banned it from young people while others want to needle kids. Why?

Why would anyone want to release the Four Horsemen of the Apocalypse? Sounds crazy, doesn't it?

I must be getting depressed, light affective disorder brought on by the onset of the Canadian winter. We are the coldest country in the world, and our prime minister is desperate to make it colder by banning and taxing energy. We in Canada, sitting on the biggest oil reserve in the world, are having to import oil. You couldn't make this up.

What do you think is happening?

Comment

1. It all seems programmed, doesn't it? The worse the economy, when you are worrying about mortgage, rent, feeding your family, and paying for heat, the less you and the population pay attention to decisions made in high places. And of course, a compliant legacy media conceals the real reason for the bad economy.

A. Exactly. That is what Mattias Desmet, the psychologist, calls the prerequisite for Mass Formation Psychosis.

October 28, 2022

Again, I have no idea what FB is doing. I wrote a post, but it seems to have vanished. Maybe if I call Klaus of Davos, KoD, the algorithm will let it through. Let me know.

Here goes. "It was the best of times, it was the worst of times, it was the age of wisdom, it was the age of foolishness," Dickens wrote in his novel *The Tale of Two Cities* about the French Revolution. History is repeating itself.

This new revolution led by KoD is called the Great Reset. The French Revolution resulted in the Reign of Terror, of mass murder, exactly like the Red Terror in Russia and the Killing Fields in Cambodia. KoD seems to be adopting the technique Mao used in the Great Leap Forward, which resulted in great hunger when thirty to sixty million Chinese died from starvation.

On orders from KoD, fertilizer was banned in Sri Lanka, which used to export food but now is starving. His acolytes have also banned fertilizer in Holland, Canada, New Zealand, and other countries. Combined with the banning of cheap and reliable energy, this winter will likely see a significant reduction in the poor and fixed income in Europe. And who knows what will happen in spring?

This outcome of the Great Reset is so obvious that it must be deliberate. This sounds like an insane statement and I hope it is. Oh well, sic transit gloria mundi; it was wonderful while it lasted. Maybe a hero will arise to give the poor, suffering humanity a chance against these overlords. Given the choice, I think I would prefer Ragnarök, the battle at the end of time, to starvation and slavery. What do you think?

Comment

1. Luckily, a few of my ancestors escaped the guillotine in France. But I was born to experience their anxiety and sense of hopelessness. With any luck, in the US the elections may help us change things without a civil war and bloodshed.

A. Given the reported incidence of contemplated suicide in the young, the sense of hopelessness seems widespread.

October 31, 2022

Help! I don't know where to turn. Medical journals are now captured by special interests and are not worth reading. You look first at who funded an article and then the position on the academic ladder of the people who wrote it. Generally, I read the ads and toss the journal.

I used to see one or two cases of gout a month. But in the last year, especially the last six months, I am seeing one or two cases a day. Many are young adults with no prior or family history.

It is strange because often the blood uric acid is normal. A gout attack was used to resolve completely with a single 50 mg prednisone pill a day for three days. Recently, it has required four or five pills. Some people even need a local injection of steroids into the painful area, which I have never done before. Maybe some are pseudo-gout, but how could you tell?

Is this a geographically isolated area? Is it by chance? What changed in the last year? Some cases with a family history or a prior attack have not had the needle, but others have, including boosters. Gout is not listed as a complication of the needle, but is it?

Ask your friends if they have seen an upsurge. If they have, maybe I should try to write it up, but the medical authorities will not like it one little bit.

Comment

That post raised a storm of observations about the not-so-hidden dangers of the needle. They included statements which seem to be true about reduced immunity, allowing dormant diseases, such as herpes and shingles, to reemerge. Also mentioned was the concept of turbo cancer, which I have heard relating to some specific conditions. These and other diseases remain to be officially confirmed.

November 3, 2022

My office in the downtown Toronto hospital is empty this morning. My offices in the suburbs and uptown are usually full. Unless they urgently need surgery, no one wants to come to downtown Toronto through the chaotic traffic occasioned by bicycle lanes with no cyclists and the endlessly blocked roads where no actual construction is taking place.

It could be worse. I remember when I first visited San Francisco, Seattle, and Portland decades ago. They were spectacular, clean, and efficient. And now! Destroyed by insane politicians. How sad!

> Gone, gone, gone with Thebes the Golden.
> Don't tell me now I didn't give you warning.

But good news. My newest book, *The Law's Delay*, has just arrived and is available online. All orthopedic surgeons deal with trauma, so we spend a lot of time in court, explaining to the judge and jury just what the injuries were and the long-term implications.

Having written more than 25,000 medico-legal reports and having testified in court as an expert witness in more than two hundred trials in Canada and the US, I have many, frequently hilarious stories. Most people will recognize some of the legendary insurance scams. I called this book a work of fiction, but you judge.

Comments

1. When I first started to come to the hospital in 1982, it used to take me twenty-five minutes to drive from Mississauga. Now, because of endless construction, it can take two hours.
2. I avoid the GTA at all costs. The traffic is terrible.

A. And public transit in Toronto is pretty terrible too.

November 6, 2022

Awake! for Morning in the Bowl of Night
Has flung the Stone that puts the Stars to Flight
(Khayyám, *Rubáiyát of Omar Khayyám*)

I forgot the clocks changed last night, so I got to the clinic at 7:00 a.m. The roads were empty. The sun was shining. A gorgeous fall day. The clinic was not open, so I walked to the local Tim's coffee shop and had a double, double and a breakfast sandwich. Normally, I avoid junk food and try for a daily eighteen-hour fast. Junk food tastes so good but makes you hungry. I tell all my patients that dieting is simple, increase the protein, decrease the carbs, and if Bill makes it, don't eat it.

Thinking of food, you will see nothing in the legacy media, but farmers all over the world are trying to warn us of the starvation to come because Klaus of Davos has banned fertilizer and is forcing the slaughter of farm animals. The followers of Klaus—Jacinda, Justine, Rutte, and the rest—are ignoring the farmers. Klaus has said that there are too many useless eaters, so presumably, this is the plan.

Stalin starved to death seven million in the Holodomor, and Mao thirty to sixty million in the Great Leap Forward. Even the totally corrupt WHO has warned that over one hundred million are at risk of starvation, but the followers of Klaus are unconcerned. I guess they feel like Stalin, one death is a tragedy; a million is a statistic.

I keep thinking that this can't be happening. But it is, and those in authority over us and the legacy media appear totally unconcerned.

But it is such a gorgeous day. So I suppose, as Walter de la Mare wrote,

Look thy last on all things lovely,
Every hour. Let no night
Seal thy sense in deathly slumber
Till to delight
Thou have paid thy utmost blessing.

—"Fare Well"

Comment

1. We are running out of diesel in the southwest US. No diesel, no trucks, no movement of goods, no food.
2. I hope you keep a stash under your bed.

A. I did once years ago when I thought that the Russians were coming through the Fulda gap that summer. But then the Polish cardinal became pope, and I knew that there would be no Russian invasion, as they would never get the tanks through Poland. Believe it or not, this time, I actually am doing a little prepping, you know, the usual—toilet paper, batteries, cigarette lighters, candles, tins of Spam, sardines, beans, thin pasta, and bags of rice. You feel like such an idiot, but why not?

November 9, 2022

Just when you think that sanity is returning, at least medically, there are moves afoot to reintroduce compulsory masking. I have never understood why these mask fanatics don't ask someone who knows about masking, like a spray painter or asbestos worker, if they would use an N95 mask for work. When they stop laughing, they will explain particle size. Universal masking was a joke and a hoax. It, along with school closures, damaged the children, and it is unclear if they will ever recover.

Something else is new. Telemedicine in Ontario is to be canceled as of December. When it was introduced at the start of the lockdown about 2.5 years ago, many doctors found it enormously useful, as they functioned perfectly well on tests and lab data. Patients naturally don't really know their own anatomy, so as an orthopedic surgeon, it never helped me much. I mean most patients have no idea where their own hip is. I am not blaming the patients; new doctors don't study anatomy as medical students and don't seem to know either. But I did find it useful in weeding out the seekers of drugs, permanent disability, orthotics, and housing, all of which plague walk-in clinics. It was very useful for close follow-up when the diagnosis was in doubt and to assess response.

Canceling telemedicine is going to result in packed clinics and parking lots, as no one wants to go to hospital emergency departments, as nursing shortages have resulted in huge wait times. No word yet of fired nurses being rehired. Some lawsuits in the US have had promising results, and the nurses might yet see justice. We live in hope.

Comment

1. It is unreal that they are canceling telemedicine. In our rural area, it has been very beneficial.
2. Telemedicine in England is very useful in dealing with simple queries and passing on the results of investigations.

A. I thought it had a very useful role and am sad to see it gone. Now we are going to see elderly people trying to use infrequent public transit or walking in the snow and ice. Relatives had to take time off work and packed waiting rooms with people coughing and spluttering in the middle of a Canadian winter.

November 11, 2022

Telemedicine in Ontario is ending as of December; the government and medical bureaucrats have decreed. They have forgotten to tell the slightly upset populace. The waiting rooms and parking lots are soon going to be awfully crowded. As everyone knows, many of the patients are elderly and infirm. So who will prevent their exposure to patients with coughs and colds?

Previously, the patients were screened before admission to the clinic by telephone consultation with docs. Using these measures, there were no known cases of transmission of the Faucian virus from the main walk-in clinic where I work. But now, if there is no screening, what will happen? Maybe nothing will happen. There was never any screening at the big-box stores, and I don't recall that they were ever targeted by the public health mob as super spreaders.

Sanity has not returned. The best engineering school in Canada has just reintroduced masking. Clearly, none of the engineers were consulted by the administration. They could have asked someone who knows about masking, like a spray painter or drywaller, if they would use a paper mask for work. When they stop laughing, they will explain to the administration about particle size. It is all so depressing that such an esteemed school should make itself a laughingstock.

And then a blithe spirit walks into the office. A girl with wanderlust. Work here, work there—Europe, the Far East, the US. Oh, to be young again! I told her of Lee Marvin's song ("Wand'rin' Star"), which was a favorite when I was young:

> I was born under a wandering star.

> Wheels were made for rolling; mules were made to pack.
> I never seen a sight that didn't look better looking back.

Or another of Kipling's poems:

> Morning waits at the end of the world,
> And the world is at our feet.

Comments

1. It is amazing how much stupidity a donation to a university can buy. Clearly, someone is interested in selling masks.
2. Your blithe must have shone like a ray of sunshine. Curiosity and imagination are rare these days.

November 16, 2022

Well, knock me down with a feather!! Kids in Canada are sick with an epidemic of respiratory infections, mainly RSV (Respiratory Syncytial Virus). What is surprising is that the public health Johnnies are surprised about this. I guess that these bureaucrats have never heard of the Hygiene Hypothesis, if you close schools and playgrounds kids are not exposed to other kids passing around common viruses. So they don't develop good immunity. When eventually exposed they may get really sick. New Zealand and Australia experienced this lockdown induced infection a year ago, and again this year. And the public health Johnnies and the children's hospitals in Canada are surprised?

And now the legacy media and some docs are screaming about masking again, especially of kids. Even if masking was of any value, kids can't use masks. They don't know how to use a paper mask, and an N95 mask doesn't fit a tiny face.

Why don't these mask fanatics ask someone who knows about masking, like a spray painter or asbestos worker if they would use an N95 mask for work. Or ask your neighborhood drywall guy if he would use a paper mask for work. When they stop laughing, they will explain about particle size. Universal masking was a joke and a hoax, and thousands knew it. So why is it being pushed? Occam's razor, i.e., that the simplest explanation is likely the correct one, suggests stupidity. But could there be other reasons? Is this just step number one in the reintroduction of mandates? Has someone got masks to sell? Just saying!

Comment

1. I refused to use a mask last time. Too many people are awake this time, or I hope so.

A. I hope you are correct, but I see an awful lot of people walking down the street on their own, wearing soiled paper masks. And hospitals are still insisting all who enter don a mask.

November 18, 2022

Wilfred Owen wrote in the desolation of WWI,

> "Strange friend," I said, "Here is no cause to mourn."
> "None," said the other "Save the undone years,
> The hopelessness."
>
> —"Strange Meeting"

Currently, the poor kids look around in dismay. Apart from the laptop class, those four-year liberal arts degree zombies who approve of the Great Reset and believe in global warming, real wages are falling. Government pensions are a giant Ponzi scheme. The recent Bitcoin fiasco has shown that there is no money. Much of the fake stuff has disappeared into the pockets of you-know-who.

The prospects are grim. Figures from Europe suggest a huge drop in fertility, presumably from the needle, so that even the comfort of the family may be denied. Brueghel's painting (google it), *The Peasant's Wedding*, showed that even in the harsh medieval times there was joy and hope.

We older people can look back on the good times.

"Those were the days, my friend,

We thought they'd never end"

- "Those Were the Days"

That fabulous decade after Woodstock with whiskey; cigarettes; wild, wild women; and the roaring boys' bravado. But then it all slowly slipped away as the Frankfurt school's long march slowly gained control and corrupted education, the media, entertainment, and politics.

It has resulted in the ludicrous situation where the James Bond villain in Davos openly boasts that more than half of the Canadian federal cabinet answers to him and not the people of Canada. Soon, by federal decree, it will become impossible to write such a statement. Only federally sanctioned "speech' will be allowed.

No wonder the pot shops are proliferating. Smoke some dope and lie around in a daze. The feds will supply universal basic income and will deliver fake food to your door.

But I suppose, while there is life, there is hope.

Comment

1. History is a great teacher, although many don't learn it. Those in power always overestimate their power and lose it when things get bad enough. There likely will be a great reset. Just not likely the one they expect. The US has always come back from seeming disasters, and, hopefully, from this too.

A. That's what we hope.

November 25, 2022

"Not to speak is to speak. Not to act is to act. Silence in the face of evil is evil," wrote Dietrich Bonhoeffer, the German pastor hanged by the Nazis in Flossenburg concentration camp on the ninth of April 1945, just one month before the end of European hostilities.

What we have seen in the last three years is only a step away with concentration—sorry, quarantine camps—still building in Australia and China.

Young men have always been scammed into wars, supposedly to protect their houses and homes. For two years they have been scammed into taking this dangerous needle. The actual number who have died of SADS, sudden adult death syndrome, remains unknown, and the outlook of long-term myocarditis is grim, as the damage to the heart is feared permanent. Young women seem to be paying an equal price, given the huge increase in miscarriage and infertility reported in Europe.

Those who have attempted to speak against this worldwide manmade disaster have been silenced and lost their licenses and jobs. Witness the current crucifixion of Peter from Texas, the world-famous cardiologist who pioneered the outpatient treatment of the Faucian virus.

But maybe things are changing. Last night, I saw two videos, 1.5 and 2 hours long, one from Europe and one from the US, detailing this apparently planned and choreographed disaster. The number of famous and respected doctors willing to give a voice was amazing.

I came to that conclusion in May 2020. Clearly, I was not alone.

Comments

1. Keep planting the seeds. It might grow into a tree of knowledge.
2. The rumbling is getting louder. Never give up.

A. I suppose, "Courage, mon ami. Le diable est mort.' Not yet, but we hope.

November 26, 2022

'But when so sad thou can'st not sadder cry,' wrote Francis Thompson. Sometimes, like T. S. Eliot, you despair that this

> valley of dying stars
> In this hollow valley

This broken jaw of our lost kingdom is what we have left our children. The collapse is all around. As Kipling wrote,

> Low among the alders lie the derelict foundations,
> The beams whereon we trusted and the plinths whereon
> we built.

We see the utter collapse of public education deteriorating into sloganeering irrelevance. Entertainment and the legacy media are simply propaganda machines that would make Joseph Goebbels proud. And politics, oh dear. "Ve haf penetrated ze kabinets and ze prime ministers." These people answer to the James Bond villain perched in Davos, and not to the public who believe they elected them.

So all is lost! Except it is not.

> In that enormous silence, tiny and unafraid,
> comes up along a winding road
> the noise of the Crusade"

(Chesterton, "Lepanto").

In spite of being fired, silenced, deplatformed, and ridiculed, the clarion call of truth is finally being heard. The cover is being torn off the machinations of the last three years.

They tried to do the same thing with H1N1 but failed, as they did not have complete media control, and heroes like Jane Burgermeister spoke out. This time they had complete control of the legacy media and the politicians and succeeded in shutting down almost the whole world for the none-too-serious Faucian virus.

But people are beginning to speak out. The untruths which led to this most heinous episode in the world's history are becoming known. God willing, Deus Vult, people will listen and act.

Comment

1. We can still speak out at present although it looks like we will lose free speech if the Canadian federal government takes control of the net, as they already have control of the legacy media.

A. If that bill passes, who knows where it will end; complete silencing of any speech, a bit like Milan Kundera's novel, *The Joke*, where the main character is jailed for telling a joke.

December 2, 2022

"May you live in interesting times." I always thought that was a quotation from Lau Tzu. It sounds like one of his maxims, which is coming true today. "Heaven and earth (or Klaus of Davos) have no pity. They regard everything as straw dogs" (*Tao Te Ching*). We certainly are living in interesting times with the funny money scam, the necessity to ban fertilizer to avert the hard-to-find global warming and the none-too-lethal Faucian virus meltdown.

I was amazed yesterday when about half the patients I saw in an uptown medical clinic were new immigrants or refugees from Ukraine. That brought this faraway war close to home. Everywhere you look in the legacy media is this constant drumbeat for war, more war. Just another $40 billion to the oligarchs or the funny money people and "we" will defeat the Russians. Good luck with that! If the Teutonic knights in 1242, Napoleon, and the Wehrmacht could not do it, I would not be holding my breath. After twenty years of war, Afghanistan was reconquered by a bunch of medieval goat herders.

And just suppose that Russia was facing a military defeat. Do you really think that they would tamely surrender? "Go gentle into that good night." Surely, even the most historically ignorant politicians understand that, given that unlikely scenario, the nukes would be unleashed.

This may be one answer to the famous paradox. Enrico Fermi, looking up at the night sky and the billions of planets, asked, "Where is everyone?" Maybe when a planet reaches a certain stage of development, unthinking politicians push it into a planet-destroying nuclear holocaust.

Or maybe as T. S. Eliot wrote,

This is the way the world ends
Not with a bang but a whimper.

Maybe, instead of nukes, the bureaucrats will continue to fund gain-of-function research to make viruses more lethal. They must be disappointed with the Faucian virus, as excess mortality data shows that the lockdown, not the virus, was the killer. This is not idle speculation as unbelievably; the US continues to fund this deadly dangerous research in Wuhan. What is wrong with these people? Is this a death wish?

Comment

1. Government old age pensions are a giant Ponzi scheme. There is, in fact, no money for pensions. So was this virus designed to clear out the pension holders?

A. That was also my initial thought, as it was so tightly stratified targeting the ill elderly. I thought it was for home consumption in China. But when one looks at the excess mortality year by year and country by country, if the objective was to kill old people, it wasn't a great success. I have heard another theory that it was a nonlethal disabling bioweapon, but again, it was not too successful at that either.

December 2, 2022

The Four Horsemen of the Apocalypse are spurring their steeds into action. The red horse of war has been provoked and deliberate expansion of that war threatens a nuclear holocaust.

Plague we have got courtesy of Faucian funding and the CCP. This one wasn't much of a plague, so they continue to fund the lab in Wuhan to try to produce a more lethal version.

The pale horse, Death, is riding among the young men. SADS (sudden adult death syndrome) they laughingly call it. We are not allowed to discuss its origin, as if people don't know. Some learned shills suggest it is due to global warming. I kid you not! Its similarity to SIDS (sudden infant death syndrome); makes one wonder if there is a connection.

Staring at the whole world is the prospect of famine. Even WHO, that fountain of truth, has predicted that, as a result of the lockdown for the Faucian virus, one hundred million are suffering what they laughingly call food insecurity. Klaus of Davos and his acolytes are closing down cheap and reliable energy and banning fertilizer and animal husbandry. It reminds one of Marie Antoinette's, "Let them eat bugs." Even in formerly wealthy countries, inflation is producing food and energy insecurity.

One wonders how much longer poor suffering humanity will put up with this. It may be longer than you think. Two hundred Bolsheviks took over Russia and held Eastern Europe in prison for seventy years.

But while there is life, there is hope. We see these incredibly brave people taking to the streets in some of the worst totalitarian regimes in the world. Will they succeed in freeing themselves? Deus Vult! God willing!

Comment

1. I am a Romanian, and we have suffered because of the communist regime in Russia, so I am not pro-Russian. But equally, I am afraid of a single major power dominating the world. Where is the "democracy" which the US promised in Libya, Afghanistan, and Iraq? Russia and the local communists imposed communism on Eastern Europe but even that fell after seventy years of misery. A form of it still exists in China although that is really just a return to the classic emperor tradition. Sadly, unless some dramatic change takes place, it looks like under the WEF the West is destined to have so-called stakeholder capitalism, which is really what Germany was in the thirties.

A. This is a horrifying thought, the Fourth Reich, but sadly, it seems quite realistic.

December 4, 2022

Telemedicine in Ontario Canada is over. It was introduced and funded by the government when the lockdown occurred and was canceled three days ago. My booked clinics are busy as ever, but the walk-in clinic is empty: the Lazarus effect we call it.

It was easy to pick up a phone for any ache or pain and get some doc sitting at home to commiserate and suggest a visit to a lab for testing or a questionable X-ray or MRI, and then a call back with the predictable negative results or possibly a suggested visit to a hands-on guy, like a general or orthopedic surgeon. Now the patient has to actually think if his symptoms are bad enough to be worth a visit. Is this good or bad? I don't know.

The free time let me look through my posts from last year. I published them in 2020 and 20021 to provide a historical record of what actually happened, as the facts were rapidly being concealed or altered by the legacy and social media. But what about 2022?

It has been exceedingly difficult, especially in Canada, for any medical professional to say anything about the needle, as there were constant threats from the authorities about losing their medical license if anything contrary to the official line was even hinted at. California is about to pass a similar law. Now Twitter has perhaps been freed from the deep state; one hopes for a tsunami of facts to emerge.

But don't hold your breath. The elf may finally be on the shelf, but the authorities and the NIH are still very much in control. No one in a university dares say anything contrary to the official line on the pain of immediate and permanent loss of research funding. Those outside academia don't understand the absolute control this gives. No research funding means no published papers and, therefore, no advancement. In effect, the end of a career. So no young scientist is going to risk it. This is why the ludicrous concept of manmade global warming persists.

For a brief moment, there was hope that freedom was coming to some benighted countries. But the tanks are on the streets of Shanghai, and the prisons in Tehran are filling up. Boethius, AD 524, wrote that "the worst misery is to have once been happy." But I don't think so. A few moments of glorious rebellion give hope that someday, we too can say, "Courage, mon ami. Le diable est mort."

Comment

1. Our health care in Canada is on the verge of collapse. My husband broke his hand at work, and we went to an emergency room. We had to wait up to twelve hours to be seen. They told us there were no nurses.

A. The hospitals fired all the nurses who did not want to take an experimental injection and refused to rehire them. It makes no sense. These women worked through the worst of the epidemic when there actually were risks, not like the current Omicron, which, if anything, is acting like a vaccine. This means the nurses and health care aides either have had the infection and are, therefore immune or have natural immunity from previous infection to another coronavirus.

DECEMBER 6, 2022

> If there were dreams to sell,
> What would you buy?
> -Thomas Lovell Beddoes, "If There Were Dreams to Sell" 1840)

I would buy Toronto in the '70s. It was a wild, free place, bursting with immigrants from Europe who had escaped the dead hand of socialism. Everyone looked forward to a bright future, to "the years that never end and know no sorrow."

It was a place of dreams; work like crazy; new ideas, new concepts, nothing impossible. And the women, who are now grandmothers, were graceful, uninhibited, independent, and wild after Woodstock (which occurred in the middle of a real flu epidemic, but no one cared). There was virtually no crime; free speech was a given; and no snowflakes; or if there were, everyone laughed at them. You could even, sometimes, trust the legacy media.

But we were so busy working and having a good time that we failed to see the creep of the long march of Antonio Gramsci and Adorno, the Frankfurt school. These faceless, joyless socialist bureaucrats gradually took over education, entertainment, and politics. I still remember the shock when they removed "shop" from school. I have no idea when they stopped Home Ed for girls.

Now I look around and weep; in Canada, there is a collapsing health care system I once thought was the best in the world. Energy prices are through the ceiling in the country with enormous reserves. In Europe, the possibility of people freezing to death in the home of the Industrial

Revolution. At the orders of the WEF, fertilizer is being banned. The WHO estimates that over one hundred million face starvation, and now, food production in the West is being further curtailed by taking farms out of production.

The oligarchs, who so admire the Chinese communists, no longer even conceal their plans for us serfs. Google "Agenda 21." Is this really what the people of the West want? And if not, how to stop it?

Comment

1. I was at the U of T in the seventies. Every Thursday, we would seek out a new immigrant bistro. The choices were many and the food excellent

A. I remember them too, all the little restaurants along Bloor and College West. There was even a Spanish place with genuine flamenco dancers from Spain who stopped by on their way to Mexico.

December 7, 2022

I have just seen a patient who came in for a shot of cortisone into his arthritic knee before going off to Panama for the winter. Lucky guy! How long will we be able to do this? The elite, of course, will continue to be able to fly anywhere in their private jets, but using the scam of global warming, we serfs will not be allowed to travel.

In the UK, they are proposing that you can travel for 15k only. I know you won't believe that but google Oxford and Cambridge where these proposals will become law. Tragically, these are the home of two of the oldest universities in Europe. So much for a liberal arts degree.

If you think that is insane, look who is still running public health in most countries. These are the people who got everything wrong in the last 2.5 years. This was a highly infectious, low-morbidity, airborne virus tightly targeted at the ill elderly and those with diabetes and obesity. Based on these facts, a medical student could point out all the errors these public health Johnnies made and continue to make. Just list them: lockdown, a CCP scam, social distancing, hand washing with toxic chemicals, Plexiglas, deep cleaning, masking, testing asymptomatic people, test and trace, ignoring diet and exercise, ignoring vitamin D, banning repositioned drugs, mandating an essentially untested needle on those who were at no risk, and on and on and on! Even a broken clock is occasionally right, but these people were consistently wrong.

Can you imagine anyone in the private sector with a litany of failures like this keeping their job?

Common sense is obviously not common to bureaucrats like this, but surely, they can read the plethora of research papers detailing their disastrous handling of this none-too-serious virus. Will there be any changes made? No sign of it so far and not likely.

Comments

1. I said two years ago that if the virus had been allowed to run its course, as happens with all flu viruses, it would just be a bad memory by now. Look at the excess deaths year by year and country by country, whether or not they did a lockdown. You can't really find an epidemic.
2. Friends of friends were given contracts to produce worthless, unnecessary PPE, ventilators that didn't work and were not required, the infamous Canadian airport app, etc.

A. The level of mismanagement was such that it is hard to believe it was just stupidity. All the little, mom-and-pop stores were closed, and the big-box stores were allowed to remain open. There was no possible scientific explanation for that.

December 10, 2022

"Do you want to go on holiday?"' A moment of panic. How do you put it diplomatically? No! Absolutely not!

I used to fly all over the world every two or three weeks for thirty years, teaching joint replacement. I wrote about it in my book, *Have Knife Will Travel.* Flying was reliable and fun with champagne and foie gras. But now? Toronto airport is the worst in the world. Go four hours ahead, line up forever here and there, maybe there is a plane or maybe later or maybe the next day. And when you come back, at least they have canceled that financial scam of the Arrive Can app. But do they still stick that thing up your nose to do the fake test and maybe get quarantined for the Mickey Mouse Faucian virus? Holiday? I'd rather shovel snow.

Even if you could travel, where would you go? Maybe Japan for Sakura time. Maybe Vietnam or Cambodia where I have never been. To return to the magnificent cities of Europe would produce a profound sense of loss as Europe is busy committing suicide.

Europe was the beacon of light in the free world, a civilization which helped lift most of the world out of abject poverty, cured diseases, abolished slavery, and gave the peoples of the world the hope that they could come from nothing and do everything.

The Enlightenment, which is being destroyed by Klaus of Davos and his oligarchs, began in 1700; the belief that an individual had worth. Now kids are taught the opposite, that they are part of a group, not individuals.

What is coming is a return to medievalism, to the masters, the oligarchs, their thugs, and the serfs. "You vil own nozink." The grim irony is that the laptop class who voted for this doesn't realize that the recent firings at Twitter show that they are serfs too. When the mines were closed, they told the miners to "learn to code." What are they going to do? Learn to do drywall?

As it is written in Hosea, 'those who sow the wind shall reap the whirlwind.'

Comments

1. The rise of Wokeism, the concept of toxic masculinity, and CRT have been pretty effective in stifling what used to be called initiative and ambition. Public education is a disgrace. It damages the children rather than teaching them anything useful.
2. School was so much fun for me many moons ago. Now, I am glad my grandson is done with school.

A. It is not only public school which is terrible. My last son, when he attended what is supposed to be a very academic school, was taught essentially no world history, none at all. He was once given an assignment, "Analyze Macbeth through a Marxist lens." I kid you not!

December 11, 2022

"Look back in anger?" I don't think so. It is more with profound regret. And yet how could it have been different? The despair of today's youth and the desolation we see around us, inhabitants of formerly wealthy countries scrambling for food and warmth. An insane response to what, in the end, was merely the bad flu, which, unlike the flu, didn't affect young people at all. SADS, sudden adult death syndrome, affecting young, fit men is certainly not due to the Faucian virus. But that was the club used to beat us into submission, into the lockdown, appropriately a term from prison. And now the scam of global warming will be used to complete the takeover.

If you google "Yuri Bezmenov," the Russian defector, speaking in 1984, you will see it has all played out exactly as he predicted. Do it! You will be amazed!

Could we have stopped it? I don't think so. It is hard to believe in a mastermind, the James Bond villain, Klaus of Davos and his cabal of young leaders. There must be other shadows behind the curtain. But who knows?

There certainly is no shortage of foot soldiers in the long march of Antonio Gramsci and Adorno and the Frankfurt school. These perhaps unwitting acolytes are in the school boards, the HR departments, the administrators, and the bureaucrats. Because no one with any ability or drive wants these jobs, the foot soldiers rise to become professors, deputy ministers, deans, joint chiefs of staff, etc.

Was it always this? I think so. Even eternal Rome couldn't keep them out. In the worst case, the end is rapidly approaching nuclear war pushed by bureaucrats; a real plague from Wuhan, which is still being funded by US bureaucrats; and starvation caused by banning energy and fertilizer.

So what should we do? I have no idea. The central governments who are producing this own the vote counting machines, the police, and the military. Look at China and Iran. But one remembers the unbelievable bravery of Tank Man in Tiananmen Square. So is there hope? Deus Vult. Maybe!

Comments

1. Nietzsche said, "what doesn't kill us makes us stronger." So we live in hope.
2. The reason Japan didn't invade the US mainland was because of the armed civilians. After Pearl Harbor, Admiral Yamamoto is reputed to have said, "I believe we have awakened a sleeping giant." The sleeping giant in the US isn't awake yet, but it's coming.

A. For the sake of the world we will leave our children, I hope. I really hope.

December 13, 2022

Gotterdammerung, the twilight of the gods or the fall of Rome! Was the West's response to the Faucian virus the equivalent?

In March 2020, in my innocence, I believed these WHO shills that the death rate was 5 percent and that this was the *big one* that we had been expecting since the Spanish flu in 1918, the one that would kill us all. But then, shortly, we learned the death rate was 0.5 percent and that kids and healthy adults were at no risk. The virus was clearly tightly targeted at the ill elderly.

Then more information began to leak in spite of censorship. The international government responses made less and less sense. When the lockdown continued and universal masking was brought in at the request of WHO during the summer of 2020 when there were virtually no deaths, it became obvious, even to someone as naïve as myself, that this had very little to do with a disease.

As anyone who has had to deal with government bureaucrats will tell you, they are utterly inept, so I am not, by nature, a conspiracy guy. I assumed, therefore Occam's razor, that the crazy response to the Faucian virus was due to stupidity. By this time, everyone knew he had funded it.

I had not paid any attention to Klaus of Davos. He did not seem real, more like a James Bond caricature. But then, his acolyte, Justine, let the cat out of the bag and drew attention to what Klaus was saying. I then heard of Event 201, held in October 2019, when they had predicted a coronavirus outbreak and had planned strategies. There then was the monkeypox outbreak, predicted long in advance to almost the week of its appearance. The WHO tried to hype that as a pandemic. But even the mask-wearing four-year liberal arts degree chaps couldn't take that obvious nonsense seriously.

Ominously, another meeting was held in October 2022 and they predict a lethal enterovirus pandemic starting in 2025. This one will kill kids and young people. This time, they plan to completely close down any dissenting voices. Laws are already being passed in Canada and New Zealand to give governments the ability to do so. I now understand why Justine, the dear leader of Canada, was so desperate to pass his internet control bill.

There is no attempt to conceal this from the public. It is, of course, not mentioned by the legacy media, who are bought and sold. This plan is presented as "just an exercise." Maybe starving in the cold and dark this winter will open a few eyes. Clearly, the oligarchs of Klaus don't care. They act as if it is game over, and they have won.

Comment

1. We feel so helpless. Even the recent US elections don't seem to have changed anything.

A. It is hard to believe that a group of oligarchs seems to be planning to take over, at the very least, all of the West. Is that what this war is all about?

December 15, 2022

'Heart of a rose, bird song at the lip, star eye, and wisdom.' I mourn the passing of Carole Aston, the wife of my oldest friend. Her husband, Peter, and I were competitive Olympic hammer throwers. He won the British Junior in 1962, and I in 1963. We have been friends since.

He was in the oil business so was constantly on the road for thirty years, as was I, teaching and demonstrating modern joint replacement surgery. We would meet in unlikely places like the Raffles in Singapore or a bar in Athens. As they lived all over the world, I would have dinner with the couple in Paris, where they were for twenty years, and other places as my schedule allowed.

I was once with them with Peter driving going into Paris. He got something in his eye so took out his contact lens. Carole leaned over from the rear seat and steered while still talking to my wife. Peter did not take his foot off the accelerator. He said, "on French roads, you must show no fear."

Two days ago, in Dorset, England, she had a massive stroke and never regained consciousness. Today, Peter kissed her goodbye, and they stopped the life support. Her spirit passed a few hours later.

A great life and a not-bad death. At least no long lingering misery. But I will miss her so.

Ave atque vale, Carole.

Comment

More than one hundred people sent condolences. It was very moving, and Peter would like to thank those who did so.

December 16, 2022

The year 2022 is almost over. In spite of the best efforts of the politicians to create one, at least no nuclear war so far. But the same buffoons are still in power, threatening war, famine, and the needle.

Civilization rises on hobnail boots (which I actually wore as a child, and I knew how to nail my own boots) and falls on satin slippers. In the West, the satin slippers are wearing out. Unbelievably, in the cradle of the Industrial Revolution, the minions of the WEF have managed to produce energy and food shortages. Obviously, this policy was not a mistake, as unrepentant, they are expropriating farms and banning fertilizer to make the food shortage worse.

Other continents appear on the ascendancy. Africa is getting rid of the Fabian Society communist rulers and the big man syndrome. The Far East, India, and Vietnam are rising. China? Who knows! This is their sixth civilization but is it rising or falling?

If you were young now, full of ambition, where would you go? Europe is collapsing, as are Australia and New Zealand. Sadly, with the recent elections, Brazil and California are becoming failed states like Venezuela. Canada is doing its best to join them.

Can the West recover? Pope Benedict said, "pruned it grows again." But if they do bring in individual carbon credits and abolish cash, it is more likely the prediction of Augustine, the Bishop of Hippo, looking across the Mediterranean at the lights going out in Rome when he said, "it is finished." And it was for one thousand years. We really hope not.

Comments

1. Some people are lost. Some of my relatives still insist on wearing a face diaper.
2. Knowing what is happening and trying to stop it on an individual basis is futile. Better just to laugh at how absurd it is and go on with your life. Eat, drink, and be merry, for tomorrow we die.

A. Mattias Desmet, the Belgian psychologist who has described the current situation as Mass Formation Psychosis, similar to Germany in the thirties, says that even one quiet, calm voice of reason might help.

December 18, 2022

My father told me to stay clear of religion and politics, but the superficially insane response to the Faucian Scamdemic inevitably draws one into the swamp.

Napoleon said that "every French soldier carries a general's baton in his pack." That was also the American dream, that a man could start from nothing and become anything he wanted. That government should stay out of the way as much as possible, and that necessary laws be fair and just. As Kipling wrote,

> Leave to live by no man's leave,
> underneath the Law.
>
> "Old Issue"

By "law: he meant English Common Law established by centuries of custom. Not the decrees of some popinjay activist judge or some elected narcissist who feels free to reinterpret the law as they see fit.

We accept that there are monstrous regimes in this world, "the dark places of the earth, full of unimaginable cruelty." But we in the West felt we had stepped away from that. But evil never really goes away. The *James Bond* series was popular because it was, in a sense, real, and the villain is back in his hideout in Switzerland.

The oligarchs who support Klaus have learned their lesson and gained control of the legacy media. But there were enough independent voices to trumpet the truth about the Faucian Scamdemic and to ridicule the attempts of WHO to declare monkeypox a pandemic.

So now the minions of Klaus in countries like Canada and New

Zealand are seeking to control the net so that only government-approved thought is allowed.

If they succeed, then it is equivalent to banning the printing press or burning the books of Averroes. And if they can abolish cash, then they have complete control, worse even than feudalism. There will be the lords, their thugs, and we serfs. If you don't follow their instructions, you can't buy anything, you can't travel, and you can't access health care.

This can't actually be happening, can it? It must be a nightmare, and we will wake up tomorrow.

Comments

1. Where in the world do you live? This rant is scary.
2. I wish it was a nightmare, but it is closer than you think. This may be our last normal Christmas.

A. The first comment sadly makes one aware that some people appear to have no idea what is actually happening. Next year, will we still be allowed to call it Christmas, or will it just be another secular government holiday?

December 23, 2022

"*Ou sont les neiges d'antan?*" wrote Francois Villon in 1480. Where are the snows of yesteryears? Was there ever a golden age? I doubt it. Hobbes (1670) was probably correct, as he was in almost everything when he said that "the life of man was nasty, brutish, and short." One dreams of the past with Pax Romana or Pax Britannica. But even then, it was as Hobbes wrote, "Covenants without the sword are but words."

Disease was a constant threat to rich and poor alike—dysentery, cholera, typhus, etc. It has been rightly said that plumbers have saved more lives than doctors. And the same is certainly true of the Industrial Revolution with the development of cheap and reliable power.

One despairs of these silly young people who want to ban fossil fuels, running around destroying works of art and gluing themselves to walls and roads. They obviously don't know that glue is made from petrochemicals.

Europe, in a suicide pact, has turned its back on cheap and reliable energy and is seemingly happy to accept that the poor will freeze this winter. Even worse, the followers of Klaus of Davos are banning fertilizer. Perhaps sheltered people like Jacinda and Justine don't understand the role of fertilizer, but surely, even they can see the result of such policies in Sri Lanka, turning it from a food exporter to starvation. The UN postulated that 150 million are in what they laughingly call food insecurity. It is hard to believe that such evil exists.

But it is almost Christmas, Christ reborn. I find it hard to think of myself as religious, but we need something to hold onto in this cesspool of corruption and evil.

"*De profundis clamavi ad te, Domine*" (Out of the depths I have cried to thee).

Comment

1. It is somewhat scary. I was talking to my Uber driver. He says he is studying robotics, and soon, drivers and all non-thinking jobs will be replaced with machines. I asked him what people will do. He said that old people are a drain on society and should go away. I now understand why Pontius Pilate washed his hands of the Jesus affair. These people are beyond saving.

December 24, 2022

> "This I ha' heard," quo' Tomlinson, "and this was noised abroad.
> And this I ha' got from a Belgian book on the word of a dead French lord."
>
> —Rudyard Kipling, "Tomlinson"

Outside the STEM field, almost everything has been said before, only better. Currently, we live in Alice's Wonderland. When Alice questions her, the Queen replies, "Why on occasion I have believed in as many as six impossible things before breakfast." That sounds like a current legacy media chap. The current crop of global warmists is like the Walrus:

> The time has come to talk of many things: . . .
> And why the sea is boiling hot—
> And whether pigs have wings.
>
> —"The Walrus and the Carpenter"

The Enlightenment, when an individual could become whatever he wanted, appears over and we are returning to feudalism. As Miguel de Cervantes wrote in 1610, "There are two families in this world, the haves and the have-nots." Currently, it is the Davos chaps, their thugs, and the rest of us poor serfs.

Looking back, we can see where it began, or at least became obvious, as the genesis was long before that. In the sixties, we became followers of

Catullus (69 BC), who wrote, “Let us live and love and pay no heed to all the tales of grim old men.” We didn’t, and now it has come to this.

All the kids were encouraged to go to daycare, masquerading as a university, where they learned nothing. Chesterfield (1770) wrote, “Knowledge of the world is only acquired in the world, and not in some closet”. (Or safe space!) Clearly, those who would ban fertilizer have never worked on a farm or grown anything.

One recognizes that the laptop class, who are the medieval equivalent of the clerisy, don’t understand that their main role will also be replaced by A.I. and that they are voting for their own destruction. Above them are the oligarchs. It took me a long time to understand what Coleridge (1830) meant when he wrote, “The motive-hunting of the motiveless malignancy.” He was describing what is emanating from Davos.

Comment

1. Merry Christmas. Perhaps the Age of Reason can be resurrected once again.

A. As Charles Dickens wrote in The Tale of Two Cities, “It was the best of times, it was the worst of times, it was the age of wisdom, it was the age of foolishness, it was the epoch of belief, it was the epoch of incredulity.” Maybe the West will recover. It succeeded against all odds at Marathon, Actium, Tours, Vienna, and Lepanto.

December 29, 2022

Do you feel like a frog in a pot? The medical clinic was not busy this afternoon, so I strolled around the neighborhood. There were an unbelievable number of video cameras attached to poles. They said, "School, slow down." But there were no schools near them. These were side streets in a very quiet residential area.

There has been no word of them being activated, but as they are solar-powered, and show the speed of the passing cars, presumably they can be switched on at a moment's notice. They must plan on doing so someday. If you put the offense speed limit at 20k, you could fine every single car.

So is this a coming tax grab, or is it something more sinister? The fifteen-minute city has been under discussion in Europe for some time, and there are grandiose plans to build such a city in Saudi Arabia. Oxford in England has just announced that they will enforce this in the next couple of years. You will not be allowed to drive out of your designated fifteen-minute zone.

You think that this can't be true. It must be some city planner's wet dream. You would think that any city council which proposed this would be booted out of office by the day's end. But in fact, there doesn't seem to be much opposition to the reintroduction of what is in reality the ghetto.

If you will submit to being locked up for two years for what for most people was the equivalent of the common cold, then the threat of global warming of 0.2 degrees in the next century will produce a paroxysm of fear.

All around the world, bureaucrats must be salivating at the thought that they too can order this. So what's next? Line up for another needle, or climb into the cattle cars for transportation to a nice holiday camp?

This can't be happening! But it is.

Comments

1. All through the virus lockdown they have been installing smart tracking, plates, and facial recognition in exactly the way they have in China.
2. If you can keep people at home, the authorities can do what they like. Imagine if we were like the Canadian truckers all on the streets. They could not stop that.

A. That's true. I remember the speech of Václav Havel in Prague. So far, the legacy media have ignored the protests. But, eventually, even STASI in East Germany could not stop the people. I was lecturing in Braunschweig, a few klicks from the border on the ninth of November 1989, the night the guards stood back, and the people pulled down the Berlin Wall.

December 31, 2022

Lambs to the slaughter! Babes in the woods! CNN or CBC reporters! You see it daily, people walking down the street, wearing a reused, soiled paper mask or lining up for a booster. So you shrug your shoulders and think that this is Darwin in action. There will be a lot fewer of them soon with the laughingly called Sudden Adult Death Syndrome affecting young men, and the tragic figures from Germany and Sweden due to the vast decrease in pregnancy and increase in miscarriage.

You wonder how they could be so naïve. And then I met a retired surgeon I have known for years. He spends his time sailing around the Caribbean when there are no hurricanes. He doesn't use the net, getting all his information from the legacy media, both print and TV. Someone had told him of one of my posts, and he was concerned I had become insane, believing all sorts of wild conspiracy theories.

It was interesting. He thought the Canadian truckers were a bunch of right-wing thugs supported by the US. He thought the Faucian virus had killed millions and that the lockdown and the needle had saved the world. He thought everyone should get a booster and kids should get the needle before going back to school. He had never heard of Klaus of Davos, the WEF young leaders, or the Minsk agreement of 2014. He thought we should send more money and guns to the Ukrainians, as they were defeating the Russians.

In the face of such beliefs, what do you say? So many medical practitioners bought into the Faucian fable and the global warming scam so completely that they cannot face the fact that they were fooled. In the country of the blind, the one-eyed man is not king, he is a pariah. If he doesn't keep his mouth shut, they will be asking him to put his feet together because they have only three nails.

So you say, "You may be right, Robin," and walk away.

Comments

1. So sad. My brother-in-law is the same. We don't bother to say anything anymore. He just thinks we are nuts if we do.
2. I know many are still fearful. I try to avoid saying anything to them.

A. You see them everywhere, the soiled-paper-mask wearers. They have completely bought into the Faucian narrative. They are like university humanities Marxist professors, impervious to facts.

January 1, 2023

Well, happy New Year. No one in the medical clinic this morning, so reflecting on the past.

When I went to St. Andrews University in Scotland, we undergrads sang a song dating back to 1267, "*Gaudeamus igitur*," which, translated, means, "Let us be happy while we are young." I also remember the Declaration of Arbroath, 1320: "As long as but a hundred of us remain alive we will fight for freedom, which no good man lays down, but with his life."

Nowadays, in schools, and universities the kids are taught nonsense, and destructive untruths, following the dictates of Antonio Gramsci and the Frankfurt school, which have taken over education, politics, the media, and entertainment. And freedom? The last two years have shown that very few value freedom.

That's not unexpected. After all, two hundred Bolsheviks took over Russia and held Eastern Europe in prison for seventy years. Klaus of Davos and his young leaders seem to have taken over the Western world and given their control of the deep state in most countries, how anyone could revolt against them is not obvious. Rationing energy has already begun, and with the banning of fertilizer, food deprivation is occurring in much of the world, and will likely arrive in the West this year.

So what can one do? In the US, the revolt seems to have begun with the taking back of the school boards, the first step in the long counter-march. "A small step for mankind."

On reflection, what I have written seems so sad. So in recompense, I quote Matthew Arnold (1880):

> To have enjoy'd the sun,

To have lived light in the spring,
To have loved, to have thought, to have done.
—"Hymn of Empedocles"

Comment

1. President Reagan said that "America is the world's last best hope. If we lose freedom in America there is nowhere else to run."

A. I hope. I have faith in "we the people."

January 2, 2023

"*Natura non facit saltus*," so wrote Carl Linnaeus (1767), the first great botanist. "Nature does not make jumps."

Sometimes it does when a giant meteor hits Earth, but most people know this to be true. When a totally new virus with a furin cleavage site suddenly appears in a city where research is being done on the same virus by someone who has been taught to insert the cleavage site, most people are able to put two and two together. Then came the furious disclaimers from those who funded this deadly and dangerous work which is of no benefit to humanity.

The legacy media, owned by special interests, hid the story. The tech industry, seemingly acting under government instructions, banned and deplatformed any attempts to debate the issue. Inexplicably, the authorities banned the use of treatments used for years and years and forced the use of treatments of dubious value at best.

This manmade disaster has led to many people questioning long-held beliefs, like the cholesterol business. I now believe that the food pyramid was written by those selling manmade foods. I tell my patients to increase the protein, decrease the carbs, and if it is manmade, don't eat it.

Without too much digging, you find interesting information. The Zika virus, which was endemic in Brazil and never produced many problems, suddenly was producing microcephaly. Except some cases didn't have Zika. A new needle was given to mothers at about the same time that this occurred. Coincidence? And how about polio in India and Africa? I am a simple surgeon so don't believe anything I say. But? But??Do your own research.

Comment

1. Something I have learned in the last couple of years is that if the media chants it, it needs more looking into. Skepticism is valid.

A. To quote Bismarck, something should only be believed when it has been officially denied.

January 6, 2023

When will this tragic comedy end? When the elderly pass on, that is sad but inevitable. All we hope is, as Longfellow wrote, that we have "left a footprint in the sands of time." But when the young die, that is another matter.

> The hand of the reaper
> Takes the ears that are hoary,
> But the voice of the weeper
> Wails manhood in glory.
> The autumn winds rushing
> Waft the leaves that are serest,
> But our flower was in flushing
> When blighting was nearest.
>
> —Sir Walter Scott, "Coronach"

Yes, yes! There has always been the odd young athlete who died suddenly of a cardiac event, but the numbers now are frightening. I do not know if professional athletes are still required to take the needle or boosters. The lesson from the *Diamond Princess* cruise ship in the spring of 2020 showed that this virus did not significantly affect healthy people, so there never was any medical indication for athletes to take it.

Similarly, there was no medical reason to compel university students to take a needle with no clear benefit and no long-term follow-up. If they wanted it, that was their choice. But mandates and compulsion were contrary to that magnificent document, the Magna Carta, signed by King

John in 1215, which stated, "To no one will we sell, to no one we will deny or delay right or justice."

To watch fit young men die on the sports fields, when as Andrew Marvell (1670) wrote, "they should be gathering their strength and sweetness into a ball to roll it through the iron gates of life." Or see the tragic figures from Europe of the drop in fertility of young women and the increase in stillbirths.

I know that many think, as H. L. Mencken, that faith is an "illogical belief in the occurrence of the improbable." But in these sad times, there is some comfort in the words, "*Agnus Dei, miserere nobis*" (Lamb of God have mercy upon us).

January 7, 2023

"Hard times produce strong men. Strong men produce good times. Good times produce weak men. And weak men produce bad times" (G. Michael Hopf, *Those Who Remain*). Trite but true, and looking at the leaders of the West, we are indeed in the weak man phase.

While we may despair of the future, a very clever lady from one of these countries in Eastern Europe wrote to me, pointing out that they have survived bad times in the past. Undaunted, they rose in rebellion against the Ottoman Empire and, centuries later, also eventually threw off the communist state.

I was lecturing in Braunschweig in 1989 when the East Germans said "enough" and the wall came down. This was in spite of the fact that one in three of the inhabitants were reported as being government informants. The heroes like Vaclav Havel in Czechoslovakia and Lech Walesa in Poland helped throw off the misery of collectivist socialism. So in Eastern Europe, they have had thirty good years.

In the West we have had almost seventy good years since the end of WWII. The good times are obviously coming to an end with the rise of the central banks, WEF, and the greens. If the relatively harmless Faucian virus could terrify the populace into giving up essentially all freedoms for two years, imagine what a really lethal virus or small nuclear bomb could do.

One sees a return to medievalism with the oligarch class and we, the serfs, allowed no animal protein, minimal heat, and travel of fifteen minutes only.

The lady from Eastern Europe acknowledges the reality of the current situation but feels that we humans have the resiliency to survive and that the good times will come again.

Comment

1. Progress is hard to achieve, and I think people are less informed and educated than they were.

A. That is my feeling also. But I now wonder when the legacy media stopped telling the truth or if they ever did.

January 14, 2023

"I never wonder to see men wicked, but I often wonder to see them not ashamed," Jonathan Swift (1740). I guess, "*plus ça change, plus c'est la même chose.*"

I looked up the definitions. A narcissist's motto is, "I am superior and need special treatment." A psychopath's is "I will take what I want and don't care how I get it." So what are we ruled by?

I always liked Thomas Jefferson's version of government:

> A wise and frugal Government, which shall restrain men from injuring one another, shall otherwise leave them free to regulate their own pursuits of industry and improvement, and shall not take from the mouth of labor the bread they have earned.

The Industrial Revolution with the development of cheap and reliable energy and chemical fertilizers in a short time lifted Europe, and then much of the world, out of poverty. Politics and religion, in some areas, slowed the development.

If you are starving, you don't care very much about your environment. If you lift people out of poverty, then they start to care about the environment. So to improve the world, you make sure everyone has cheap and reliable energy and chemical fertilizer. Inexplicably, the Davos overlords are endeavoring to ban both. Even the suborned "young leaders" of Klaus must know in their heart of hearts how evil and destructive these policies are.

So are they psychopaths or narcissists or something else?

Comment

1. They are evil incarnate and, thereby, both psychopaths and narcissists.

A. I suppose history will judge, but sadly, the winners write history, and things are not looking good for the common people.

January 18, 2023

"That one may smile, and smile, and be a villain" (*Hamlet*, Act 1, Scene 5). We are currently seeing just such a replay in Davos.

I never ever thought I would waste my time thinking about politics. I despised those I knew at university who were members of political clubs. These now are the people running governments. I always felt that those who wanted to rule and sit in judgment over us were the people who should never be allowed to do it.

People outside the licensed professions have no idea how rigid the control of the licensing bodies is. Currently, the College of Psychologists of Ontario is trying to silence Jordan Peterson, the world-renowned public intellectual. Doctors also have to answer to hospital administrators and government ministries of health and if you are university, deans, and the controllers of research funds.

It was for these reasons that the medical profession was amazingly silent about the Faucian virus. The data from the *Diamond Princess* cruise ship showed that the virus was fairly innocuous. It was the anti-scientific crazed response to it that severely damaged the middle class, threw thousands into poverty, and resulted in the starvation for millions.

Sadly, it seems that even that was not the main tragedy. The fear is the long-term effect of the needle on immunity, autoimmunity, resistance to neoplasm, and fertility. The data from Europe has shown a drastic reduction in fertility. For the other fears, we will have to simply wait and pray.

Comment

1. The virus became the perfect political weapon to complement the climate change hysteria, and the legacy media is fully on board.

A. The legacy media is simply the organ grinder's monkey dancing to their master's tune.

January 20, 2023

"Put not your trust in princes!" (Psalms 146). Especially those currently in Davos, plotting our future with no cheap and reliable energy, no travel, no food except bugs, and complete government censorship of all media. The future for our kids looks terrible.

And then a lady I haven't seen in years dropped by. When the weather is good, she and her husband walk the pilgrim routes in Europe like the Camino de Santiago in Spain.

I remember forty years ago, sitting beside her at the sharp end of a plane, drinking mimosas, as it lifted off from Toronto airport into the sunshine on the way to Korea. I had a lot of surgery planned, and she was my scrub nurse and spoke Korean. On that trip, one day in Seoul, we did a knee replacement in four separate hospitals. The last one was a twenty-four-year-old girl with a smashed knee. The knee I put in lasted twenty-three years. I know because the son of the man who asked me to do it told me when he revised it.

We did a lot of surgery in the Far East. Once in Thailand, we did a knee replacement in front of a large audience. For that, usually you need at least a couple of cameramen. That day, there was one guy with a little camera, a smaller monitor, and a step ladder. He was superb. The Thais asked the nurse what she wanted to take back to Canada. "We'll take the cameraman," she said.

Her long black lustrous hair is now white, but she is the same magnificent clever woman. We talked about the feeling while walking the labyrinths in Europe, especially Chartres Cathedral. It makes one feel that there is still hope in the world.

Comment

1. Beautiful experiences create beautiful memories. Sadly, Fascism is alive at Davos.

January 28, 2023

"This will be my last visit." A ninety-year-old man I have been treating for back pain for three years told me that this morning. He was always fit, vigorous, well-dressed, and cheerful, determined to extract as much gaiety as possible from the life that was left. This morning, he looked old and tired. He could see the gates of death opening for him. His wife of sixty years was also present and silently weeping.

I believed him. Some people just know. I gave him his treatments and we embraced for the first and last time. A brave man facing his death with equanimity. I only hope I show the same courage when my time comes.

And then the next patient is a young girl who wants to be a doctor but can't get into medical school in Canada. Decades ago, a couple of useless economists wrote a government report, saying there were too many doctors in Canada, so the government reduced the number of places in medical schools. The economists clearly didn't know that an aging population needs more health care.

So where should she go? If she trains in England, she will never get back into Canada and is condemned to work in Europe, a continent committing slow suicide with no energy, no food, and a determination to provoke WWIII. I suggested the Caribbean as, from there, she will finish her training in the US and can be licensed there. Again, she won't get back into Canada, but that is also busy following Europe into oblivion.

When I was young, there were endless choices.

> "Morning waits at the end of the world,
> And the world is at our feet."
>
> -Rudyard Kipling, "The Gipsy Trail")

But now, where would you go? Florida? Singapore?

Comment

1. My nephew went to UCC in Ireland for medical training. He was extremely lucky to get a residency in Canada, but it was very tight.
2. Talk her out of being a doctor.

A. In theory, they can get back into Canada, but it is very, very difficult for graduates from non-Canadian schools to acquire a medical license. Medicine is now so tightly government-controlled that effectively doctors are becoming bureaucrats. So I told my son to be an engineer.

January 29, 2023

Snow again! Where is the promised global warming? Canada is statistically the coldest country in the world, but our dear leader wants to make it colder.

As many, but sadly not all, are beginning to realize that they were fooled by the response to the none-too-serious Faucian virus, the elites in Davos are again ramping up the global warming rhetoric with boiling oceans, rain bombs, etc.

How can anyone take these people seriously? They fly to conferences all over the world in their private jets, flown by pilots who have not had the needle. They congratulate themselves on saving the world by keeping the wretched of the earth poor and starving by banning cheap power. They impoverish formerly rich countries with ridiculous legislation and debt. They push for WWIII which none of them will ever fight.

They plan on inserting mRNA into all domestic animals. Remember those thousands of dead cattle the legacy media claimed were due to global warming! It has reached the stage where one puts on a tin hat and wonders about all these dead chickens.

It is no longer just theoretical. In Edinburgh, Scotland, they have banned meat in school lunches, doubtless to be replaced by Bill's bugs. The fifteen-minute cities are coming online (google Oxford). You will be forced to remain in your ghetto.

We felt some hope when, in New Zealand, the acolyte of Klaus of Davos was forced to step down. Sadly, the replacement seems worse, mandating the needle, which is now recognized as doing far more harm than good.

You sit back and think this can't actually be happening. I thought Revelations was magic—mushroom-induced nightmare.

Comment

1. There is some very interesting research being done on magic mushrooms.

A. So I heard. In John Hopkins, I believe. What is interesting is that that classic shamanistic dream seems common. Does Yggdrasil, the tree of life, actually exist?

February 4, 2023

"Sit down and shut up!" It was hilarious, listening to one of these famously short-tempered business coaches answering a student who asked about the effects of rising sea levels on future economies.

"Biggest scam the world has ever seen," he said. "I only wish I had thought of it first. If it was true, do you think that the financial institutions in the US and London would give you a forty-year mortgage for a beachfront property that these charlatans say will be underwater in ten years?"

He is right! Actuaries are highly paid, dry, emotionless, enormously clever people whose job it is to assess risk. They are not in the business of making mistakes. Laughably, these hypocritical celebrities who bellow about global warming buy beachfront mansions. It is freezing in Toronto this morning. I wish global warming was real, but it feels like we are actually entering a grand solar minimum.

Who knows what to believe nowadays. The so-called experts are either government bureaucrats or are people funded by organizations or foundations with vested interests, usually something to sell.

I had a very entertaining, highly educated Afghan lady in my clinic yesterday. She knows the history of that Graveyard of Empires and the sorrow of Balkh, the mother of cities. She is in the travel business so flies frequently and has just come back from that country. She says the airport in Kabul is a lot more efficient and hassle-free than Toronto. Interestingly, she told me that her sister, who runs a school for girls in Kabul, has not had any official interference. True or not! I don't know. Currently, I believe what Bismarck, the Iron Chancellor of Germany said, "That something should only be believed when it has been officially denied."

There is still no official cause for SADS, sudden adult death syndrome, which sounds a lot like SIDS, sudden infant death syndrome. I never thought of that before but is there a connection? There are laughable reasons given like global warming or eating eggs. I hear someone is now in the business of producing fake eggs, and surprise, surprise, one of the biggest egg-producing plants in the US has just burned down. I am sure it is completely coincidental.

Comment

1. Until recently, there were articles on the net from scientists who were saying that, based on the sun's activity, a new ice age is coming. These articles are now almost impossible to find.

A. It is called a Milankovitch cycle. Information is there from very reputable scientists but is difficult to find. One does not want to laugh, but if anyone actually believes in manmade global warming, I have a bridge in Brooklyn for sale.

February 6, 2023

Awake! for Morning in the Bowl of Night
Has flung the Stone that puts the Stars to Flight
- Omar Khayyám, *Rubáiyát*).

There is good news on the horizon. The UK has just joined the Nordic countries in banning the needle in the under fifties. Surrounded as we are by the monsters coming out of the closet in Davos bringing war, famine, disease, and destitution, any sliver of good news is wonderful.

I just listened to a podcast featuring Robert Malone, the developer of mRNA. He, with a band of fearless docs and scientists like Geert, Knut, and Sukharit, has been trying to warn the world for a couple of years. They have done so in the face of extreme opposition from the legacy media, big tech, and all these three-letter government agencies.

Malone went through in detail how the relatively harmless Faucian virus was used as a weapon to induce Mass Formation Psychosis, as termed by Mattias Desmet, the Belgian psychologist. He points out that the government "nudge" agencies were using sophisticated psychological techniques (PsyOps) to terrify the populace into accepting clearly nonsensical orders, such as closing mom-and-pop stores and leaving big-box stores open and closing schools for a disease that didn't affect kids.

So the banning of the needle in Europe is a welcome step toward sanity. If only North America would follow suit.

And wouldn't it be wonderful if we could ban green energy and remove the followers of Klaus of Davos from positions of authority, as they clearly answer to him and not to the people who supposedly elected them?

Oh, well. Dream on.

Comment

1. May truth prevail.

A. Immanuel Kant said the truth will out. But that was before the reach of big tech.

February 8, 2023

"You only have power over people as long as you don't take everything away from him. Once you take everything, he is no longer in your power ." (Alexander Solzhenitsyn, *The Gulag Archipelago*).

The current worldwide disaster is because governments still have something to take away from us. For the licensed professions, it is the loss of license, which is why there was never any outcry about the abandonment of Western medicine and the acceptance of the lockdown and then an untested gene therapy.

For many, it was their jobs and ability to travel, and for students, it was to attend university. But inflation and the destruction of cheap and reliable energy will put an end to jobs in food production and manufacturing in the West. So all is doom and gloom as the monsters in Davos reveal their plans to dominate the poor and suffering humanity.

But then we remember Lech Walesa scrambling over the gate in Danzig and the Berlin Wall coming down. So maybe, as Bernard Shaw wrote about Pharsalus, "The impossible came to pass; the blood and iron on which ye pin your faith fell before the spirit of man." Spring is coming and with it maybe freedom.

Comments

1. Stay positive. Stay loud. The truckers and the farmers have already started to fight the erosion of our rights and freedoms. Hopefully, others in Canada will wake up.
2. Every day, more of their evil is revealed. There has been an enormous transfer of wealth from the ordinary people to the elite

on a conveyor belt of deceit and corruption. You have inspired me to get involved in my community and add my voice to the growing number of those seeking positive change in our part of East Tennessee.

A. As Yogi Berra said, "It isn't over til it's over."

February 11, 2023

"Whence comest thou, Gehazi, . . .
in ermine and in gold?"

-Kipling, "Gehazi".

For those who know the Book of Kings and the prophet Elisha, that quote is entirely appropriate for the current influencers in world affairs. If you don't know, google it.

Those in large part responsible for the disastrous response to the none-too-serious Faucian virus are being awarded wealth and honors; some in the UK with knighthoods, and others with gold-plated pensions.

In the past, none of those responsible for the nightmares of the Holodomor, the Killing Fields of Cambodia, or the starvation of the Great Leap Forward paid any price. The Nuremberg Trials have never been repeated for the Gulf of Tonkin, the weapons of mass destruction, etc. But maybe, just maybe, justice is coming for the virus Scamdemic.

In the US, nurses who were fired for refusing the possible anti-fertility needle have won some court cases for compensation, and some even for being forced to take the needle against their wishes. Sadly, these were out-of-court settlements, so they don't establish a precedent.

In Thailand, some relatives of the king were severely injured by the needle. They have listened to Sucharit Bhakdi, one of the heroes of this disaster who has been warning the world about the potential problems with the needle for a couple of years. The Thai government is seeking legal recompense.

Even in Europe, while I find it hard to believe, some senior elected officials have been charged over procurement and mandates of the needle. Some senior EU officials are also under investigation.

So maybe, just maybe, there will be justice for these damaged and dead young men and these young women having difficulty conceiving.

Addendum. I got a warning from FB that this post was unacceptable. I never know if they have taken it down completely or just shadow-banned it, so I asked people to confirm if they could see it. Many did, and I am very grateful. I knew all about censorship in Eastern Europe before the wall came down and in other bastions of freedom like Cuba and China, but I never expected it in the West. The sorrow of it.

"Ye mountains of Gilboa let there be no dew upon you . . . nor fields of offerings."

(2 Sam. 1:21).

February 15, 2023

Does pure evil exist? Who knows! but look at the major industries of medicine, food, education, war, and entertainment.

Everything I was taught in medical school about diet was wrong. I was told animal fat kills, so I used trans fats for the next forty years. I was told red meat and eggs are bad and cereal good. Then came the Faucian virus. The data from the *Diamond Princess* and the US aircraft carrier showed it was about as lethal as the flu, and essentially, no healthy person under seventy was at risk.

The response of continued lockdown, masking, and then mandating an experimental gene therapy was contrary to all Western medicine, tradition, and common sense. The information being fed to the public was so obviously untrue that my belief system was profoundly altered, and I began to question everything.

I found believable information on the net from sources as diverse as a South African GP, world-famous docs, and an Irish engineer whose simple and penetrating analysis of actual government statistics showed that no intervention had any positive effect on the virus. This was glaringly obvious by May 2020, and yet, the craziness continued and still does in some countries.

So if the government policy on this is wrong, then what else is wrong? Ivor, the Irish engineer, analyzed the data on the actual challenges of our time, —diabetes, cardiac disease, and obesity. He showed that all government advice on diet was as bad as their advice on the virus and that everyone should take more medication.

I now believe diet is simple: increase the protein, decrease the carbs, and if it comes in a box, don't eat it. Avoid seed oils that were manufactured originally as an engine lubricant. Cook with butter, lard, and olive or avocado oil. If the vegetable grows above the ground, eat more; if below the ground, eat less. Fruit juice is pure sugar. Read the sugar content of modified fruit; some are just candy.

Remember, I am a simple surgeon, and my information source is an engineer, so don't take anything I say too seriously. But those producing the government food tables that are poisoning the populace must have known what they were doing. Stupidity is not a good excuse. So the question of evil arises.

February 17, 2023

Just got a message from FB telling me I have been banned. I knew I was being shadow-banned, but this looks complete. It is hardly a surprise. Anticipating this, I have collected all my posts of 2022, documenting the tragic mismanagement last year. I plan on possibly publishing these in book form. If anyone can see this, perhaps suggest a title like *Plandemic-Scamdemic*, or *The Collapse of the West*, as the Davos gang seem to be morphing the virus lockdown into a permanent global warming lockdown.

Oh well. The Enlightenment was great while it lasted; sic transit gloria mundi. Governments around the world are busy banning free speech. As Dowson wrote,

> They are not long, the days of wine and roses:
> Out of a misty dream
> Our path emerges from a while then closes
> Within a dream.

There are still heroes. In the middle of the misery of the Canadian winter (where is the promised global warming?), I saw a big, strapping girl in my clinic yesterday. She works as a diamond driller in a mine in the Yukon. To get there she says catch a company plane in Edmonton and fly two hours due north. Forty below, she says is like spring. When the wind blows, it is more like 60 below. This is one tough girl. But she says her job is a lot easier than the roughnecks in the oil fields.

It is sobering to think that we live such an easy, cushioned life because people like her are up north, breaking themselves in two. These heroes don't get the credit and admiration they deserve.

People gave me all sorts of advice on how to get unbanned, and I am very grateful. I wish we lived in a world without censors.

February 18, 2023

Yesterday was like a dream. There was freezing rain in the morning, so all the trees and shrubs were coated with ice. The setting sun made the branches and tiny icicles hanging from them glisten like diamonds-magical. Thinking Walter de la Mare,

> Look thy last on all things lovely,
> Every hour. Let no night
> Seal thy sense in deathly slumber.

Also had a writing session with my coauthor and friend, Edna Quammie. Hard to believe that we met in 1972, as described in our first book, *The Big House*, where we described those wild days after Woodstock, which changed how we viewed the world. The poor kids nowadays, terrified of "me too," have no idea of the fun and frolic their grandparents had.

Edna and I thought we had exhausted the tales of the malfeasance of big pharma in our third book in the *Qian Choi* series, *Rogue Pharma*, which will soon be available in audiobooks. But as more details continued to leak out, it became obvious that an additional book of revelations, mayhem, and revenge was required.

It is interesting trying to write in such a way as to avoid being canceled by an increasingly authoritarian government and big tech. We are more careful now than we were even two years ago, so from our actions, the censorship is actually worsening, not improving.

February 20, 2023

As usual, Shakespeare got it right in the tragedy of *King Lear*:

> The weight of this sad time we must obey,
> Speak what we are told, not what we ought to say.
> The oldest hath borne most; we that are young
> Shall never see so much nor live so long.

In some parts of the world, young men seem to have given up. In China, I believe they call it the "lie down" movement. In Japan, they stay home and play video games. Why? I don't know.

The same thing is happening in the West, but here the cause is obvious. In school, if a boy acts like a boy, he is disciplined and drugged with Ritalin. The "teaching" is pathetic, mostly simply the indoctrination of obvious untruths. Shop, where something useful used to be taught, is banned. Universities are worthless. Poorly educated, semi-literate professors let people graduate with an arts degree without reading Shakespeare or Kit Marlowe.

Normal male activity is called toxic masculinity. Ambition and drive are discouraged. Promotion in academia or any government-run or -influenced position is no longer based on competence. Even the military in the West has been downgraded to such an extent that young men no longer wish to serve. Why should they when leaders, such as Justine in Canada, do not look at the nations they serve as nations but post-national states, simply a piece of real estate to be run by agencies, such as WHO and WEF?

What is even more strange is that these leaders seem determined to provoke WWIII. Maybe the global warming scam is not giving them enough control and a really big war is required. Who would have thought that *Brave New World* and *1984* were not novels but playbooks?

Maybe it is not that bad. Spring is coming. Civilization has survived worse.

February 24, 2023

Mass Formation Psychosis is the term coined by Mattias Desmet, the Belgian psychologist, to describe the insanity of the worldwide response to the none-too-serious Faucian virus and the even greater and potentially infinitely more destructive myth of manmade global warming. Desmet believes, as did Pastor Niemöller (google him), that a few sane voices raised in protest can make a difference and can calm the lynch mob. So why is there a deafening silence? Government and big tech have insidiously worked their way into every aspect of our lives: diet, speech, education, entertainment, etc. In medicine, one of the fundamental principles is informed consent. But a patient can only give informed consent if he/she is informed about the cost/benefit of the treatment.

Since the advent of the Faucian virus in most Western countries, incredibly, doctors have been forbidden to express any opinion contrary to the official government diktat. In effect, treatment is mandated by the government. In care homes in the UK, shortness of breath was assumed to be due to the Faucian virus and was treated with morphine and Midazolam. Breathing soon ceased, which solved the problem.

If this is seen by governments as a success, then in the future, if you have a medical problem, you will access a government site on your phone, type in your symptoms, and the algorithm will prescribe you pills which will be delivered by drone. No need to leave your fifteen-minute city (ghetto). If you are anxious, some dope will also be delivered, and maybe your ration of fake food and Bill's bugs.

A year ago, the concept of a fifteen-minute city would have been unimaginable. But now it is occurring all over England. It is being brought in against the will of the people. Is this the future or can it be reversed? I can't think of any collapsing civilization which recovered. So are we on the way to Gehenna? I hope not.

Comments

1. Martin Niemöller: "I did not speak out —— and then they came for me—and there was no one left to speak for me." Another good read is *The Banality of Evil* by Hannah Arendt.
2. People seem to be waking up, but it has almost reached a cult stage where "you are the enemy if you dare think otherwise." Just like Germany in the thirties.

A. The widespread acceptance of brainwashing or Mass Formation Psychosis is really quite frightening. Hannah was right, just a few decades early. She would recognize exactly what is happening—the tyranny of the bureaucrats.

February 25, 2023

Snowing heavily, so the clinic is empty (where is the promised global warming?), so time to think.

What is the purpose of a university? I have been associated with them all my life and have seen them change beyond all recognition.

When I went to St. Andrews University in the '60s, there were two distinct classes, the scholarship boys like myself who were there for the best degree possible in the shortest possible time, and the leisure class, like the prince royal and his bride. For them, the university was a sort of finishing school, not to be taken seriously.

Then only about 10 percent of the young people went to university and the leisure class was quite small. But then politicians began to expand the number of 'universities' and now more than 50 percent of young people attend.

To accommodate this huge influx, universities changed. Standards dropped precipitously, and Mickey Mouse courses called 'studies' were introduced. The teachers of these courses were all but illiterate themselves, the blind leading the blind if you will. Even the STEM fields are becoming corrupted, as demonstrated by the Faucian virus scandal. Effectively, universities have become daycares, prolonged adolescence.

So what to do? Obviously, all liberal arts and most universities should be closed or converted to technical schools. But how do you change the prospective employer's demand for a four-year degree? AI is replacing the lower end of white-collar jobs. This is obvious any time you go near a bank. The global warming crowd, egged on by the WEF, by banning reliable sources of energy, is deindustrializing the West, so will there actually be any jobs left in the next twenty years?

The answer to the WEF seems to be to sit in your fifteen-minute city (ghetto), smoke dope, eat Bill's bugs delivered by drone and join the metaverse. Fortunately, the metaverse, which was launched with great fanfare, seems to have disappeared, so maybe there is still some hope for humanity.

Comment

1. I am not sure taxpayers should be paying for public education as it now stands. Here in Oregon, it is extremely expensive and subpar. This year, they introduced "Equitable Grading," lowering the standard even more and reducing what was left of student motivation.

A. I agree. I don't believe public schools work anymore. I think they should be replaced by charter schools and technical schools.

March 1, 2023

Shoveling snow and thinking, What are the problems facing humanity? It is certainly not global warming. Contrary to reports in the legacy media, extreme weather events are not increasing, and no one has been displaced by rising oceans. Those oligarchs who fly to meetings in exotic locales in their private jets and constantly lecture us on rising sea levels buy beachfront mansions. Oh well. Hypocrisy is hardly news!

Problems vary. For the poor little children slaving away in the mines in Africa to produce cobalt for the batteries for green vehicles, it is getting some food at the end of the day. The housewife searching for twigs or animal dung to make a fire to cook the family's evening meal; it would be a cheap, reliable energy unavailable because the oligarchs bribe the leaders of these countries not to build coal plants. India and China are building coal plants daily to lift their people out of poverty and despair.

If you are starving, pollution is the least of your problems. People begin to worry about pollution when their annual family income exceeds $7,000.

If you are an academic, work for the government, or a woke corporation, the only expression allowed is the mandated opinion. You are expected to believe and mouth what you know to be untrue.

But in spite of shadow-banning and censorship, the net does provide information otherwise almost impossible to get. People are becoming aware of the craziness of the response to the none-too-serious Faucian virus. Almost without exception, the whole world followed the authoritarian CCP lockdown. The question is did the CCP actually lock down themselves, or was it a Potemkin village? We know most of the videos from China of people dropping dead in the street were fake. Possibly concerned about a falling population, they wisely did not let their own people take the mRNA needle.

So put on your tin hat! Are we living in the matrix, or have we just lost WWIII?

March 3, 2023

I am a cyborg. I realized that yesterday. Elon Musk had said that years ago, pointing to his cell phone, but I didn't realize it until I couldn't find mine.

My secretary and I had wasted the whole morning studying for and taking the mandatory exams for my annual reappointment to the teaching hospital. It had absolutely nothing to do with medicine. Not being closely acquainted with the woke modern world, I could not possibly have passed it on my own. She was able to answer the questions, so I am reappointed for another year. I don't know why I bother. It doesn't seem worth it.

So I was late for my afternoon clinic. When I reached for my cell phone to explain to the second patient, I realized I didn't have my phone. A moment of blind panic ensued. I realized I couldn't function without my electronic device, the true definition of a cyborg.

In this clinic, at least half the people don't speak much English, which is increasingly common in some parts of Toronto. With my cell phone, I can show them the problem, and they can find it on their phone in their own language. Without a cell phone, it is impossible to run a clinic like this. The clinic phoned my secretary, who got a taxi and brought mine and saved the day. Heart be still!

I find it difficult to think of life without it. If you are bored, google "Philosophy in Five Minutes" and listen to the wisdom of Seneca or Kierkegaard. Who needs to go to a liberal arts university? The lectures on the phone are far superior to some struggling teaching assistant. If it is a long drive, you can listen to a Jordan Peterson or Joe Rogan podcast.

It seems to me that university humanities professors are obsolete. And increasingly, I am beginning to think a lot of doctors are also. The speed of change is breathtaking.

Comment

1. Don't give up teaching. Someone has to help the kids out of Plato's cave. The Faucian virus fiasco resulted in some waking up and leaving, but an awful lot remains behind.

A. Sadly, the left-behinds in the cave are seen every day, walking down the street with these futile, soiled paper masks.

March 5, 2023

It is what we called in Scotland 'a soft morning'. The snow is piled high making driving through the side roads difficult, but it feels like spring. As Kipling wrote,

> Robin down the logging-road whistles,
> 'Come to me!'
> Spring has found the maple-grove,
> the sap is running free.
>
> "The Flowers"

For those of us who came to Toronto in the early '70s, there is a lingering sense of the magic, a city with new immigrants from Europe escaping from the tyranny of socialism. There was the belief that you could do what you wanted, be what you wanted, work like crazy, make money, and make love. And the women were proud, free, and utterly independent.

But now, the freedom, the magic, all gone, "gone, gone, gone with lost Atlantis." The stultifying dead hand of socialism, from which we thought we had escaped, has come back with both hands around the throat of the whole West, especially the Anglo world.

That bold Métis woman who helped organize that awe-inspiring, peaceful Canadian trucker protest, which succeeded in lifting the anti-scientific, ludicrous, destructive mandates, is facing ten years in jail. Martial law was declared, bank accounts frozen, and trucks confiscated. Tragically, not a single leader in the free world raised a voice in protest.

These so-called leaders appear to answer to Klaus of Davos and not the people who elected them. Using the ludicrous scam of global warming, they are destroying reliable energy, manufacturing, car ownership, travel, and food production. Even more alarmingly, they are forcing gene therapy with no long-term data onto not only the people but also the livestock. The people in Prague in 1968 must have felt the same despair when the tanks rolled in. But about twenty years later, the Berlin Wall came down, bringing freedom with it.

So what are we looking at? Twenty years of increasing misery, WWIII, or freedom? In Scotland and New Zealand, the Gauleiters of Klaus have lost office. On a morning like this, you think there is hope.

March 8, 2023

"Truth will out," said Immanuel Kant. Really! Who would ever believe that? And yet in the UK, a courageous ghostwriter has just released the files of one of the more important Faucian disaster government shills. And wonder of wonders, a major newspaper, *The Daily Telegraph*, has published some of the details.

By May 2020, it was obvious to anyone with the slightest medical knowledge that this was a Scamdemic; that healthy people under sixty were at virtually no risk, kids neither got sick nor transmitted the virus, social distancing was silly, Perspex was worse than useless by slowing air exchange, school closures were child abuse, etc. So why was an untested experimental gene therapy mandated for all?

Those who tried to point out the reality were, at the minimum, shadow-banned or censored, and doctors were threatened with the loss of medical licenses.

I thought that the old saying that "dogs bark, but the caravan passes" was true, so to leave a written record of what actually happened, I published my posts in book form or added some romance and called it fiction, the *Qian Choi* series, most recently, *Rogue Pharma*, soon available in audiobook.

This release of information in the UK is spectacular. Of course, the lady is being attacked by all the usual media shills, including the famous Channel 4 zealot who ignominiously tried to attack Jordan Peterson.

Other cracks are appearing in the dam of misinformation. A Cochrane report has confirmed what everyone in the skilled trades knew, that masking was worthless. Numerous publications now confirm that the needle is of no particular value and potentially damaging. Sadly, in the fiefs run by the disciples of Klaus of Davos, such measures are still being pushed.

Mahatma Gandhi said that, "if you vote for a fool, that's what you get." But looking around, does foolishness really explain the events of the last few years?

Comments

1. I am so pleased the truth is beginning to come out. Every layman high school grad knew this was a hoax. Those who usually don't think were scared into obedience.
2. This was not foolishness. It was pure evil.

March 10, 2023

Great day yesterday. Fascinating patients; one of them was an old professional middleweight boxer who had more than one hundred fights. It wasn't the fights that were the problem; he had been knocked off his motorcycle. We call these donor cycles, as that's where the organs for transplant come from. The best rider in the world is at the mercy of the biggest fool with the smallest car. When I was a boy in Scotland, we were allowed to see very little TV, just Shakespeare's plays, Westerns, which my father regarded as old-fashioned European miracle plays, and fight of the week from America, all these fabulous middleweights like Dick Tiger.

The man with him was someone I knew, one of the few genuine stonemasons in Canada. I always admired the men who created these wondrous medieval buildings in Europe. I had always wanted to be one, but surgeons end up with arthritis in their thumbs.

Then there was a girl with a bad back. She had fought MMA but had hurt her back in a car accident. Her treatment had been dreadful. She had strained her back, but they told her it was a serious injury, that she must stop exercising, rest, and see them frequently for hot packs, ultrasounds, massages, and manipulations. When I saw her first she was heavy, weak, stiff, depressed, and hopeless. I gave her some local anesthetic blocks and sent her to yoga and Pilates. She is so much better, brighter, lighter, and hopeful. After two years of worthless treatment, she has a long way to go. She needs to get back to the gym with the hard-ass fighters.

And then a former pro football player I have known for years; a calm, clever, sensible man. He is fed up with Canada and going south. I gave up my Florida medical license years ago. He encouraged me to see if I could reactivate it. Dream on! It's snowing again outside. Sarasota would be so nice!

Comments

1. I live in the US now. I need my left knee revised. Come on down!
2. I look out of the window at the piled snow and dream of Sarasota.
3. You sound more positive. Is it the promise of rebirth and the lightness of summer?

A. In Canada, with the long winter, I think we all suffer from some degree of Light Affective Disorder. I used to have a place in Longboat Key. I wish I still had it.

March 15, 2023

Interesting morning. The first patient was a Polish man with acute sciatica. It is March break, and he is taking his kids south to Key West to see where Hemingway lived. I gave him some paralumbar blocks a couple of days ago, and now at least, he is standing straight. I repeated them this morning, as this afternoon he will be facing the misery of Toronto airport with its uncaring bureaucrats and an utterly incompetent airline.

I hope he makes it. Hemingway was one of my favorite authors. In this age of illiterate professors and melting snowflakes, one would never admit having read great stories like *The Short Happy Life of Francis Macomber* or *Across the River and into the Trees.*

How times have changed. I grew up reading *De Bello Gallico*, Caesar's war diaries, and Rudyard Kipling's India. I was once at a dinner party in New Delhi and was talking to the general who commanded the Indian forces in the Indo-Chinese war in 1962. He told me Kipling was the greatest Indian poet. "But he was English," I said.

"Nonsense," said the general. "He was born and brought up in India. Of course, he was Indian." I thought then and still think, what a magnificent worldview, that we were all going forwards together into a bright future.

And then you think of the monsters crouching in Davos, threatening the world with war, famine, and the abolition of cheap and reliable energy. I think I hope the world is waking up to this evil and that it is not too late.

Comment

1. I have been in the hotel where Hemingway liked to stay in Havana.

A. The Polish man had taken his kids there the year before. How magnificent.

Envoi

How will this episode end? Firstly, was it a disaster? That now seems clear and indisputable. It was not the manmade virus, which was the problem, it was the response to it. If there had been no PCR testing, no one would have known there was a rogue virus on the loose. In reality, there was no epidemic or pandemic.

Secondly, why was the response so disastrous? One is always tempted to ascribe all manmade disasters to stupidity, but this was so egregious, that that is not a tenable explanation. So the underlying reason remains obscure.

Thirdly, will we ever know the truth? This is the end of year three, and there is no uniform consensus as to why the world acted in this calamitous fashion. The temptation, or perhaps the reality, is to see this as simply an episode in the collectivization of the world, an opportunity to accustom the populace to obey nonsensical rules, thus paving the way for *1984* or the *Brave New World*. We hope not. But in the end, we will simply have to wait and see.

Published Books

Technical

The Technique of *Total Hip Replacement*
The Bone Implant Interface

Autobiography

Have Knife Will Travel

Current Events

Journal of the Plague Year (2020)
Plague or Pseudo Plague 2021
The Law's Delay

Novels

To Slip the Surly Bonds of Earth
Book 1 *About the Breaking of the Day*
Book 2 *Upon the Further Shore*
Book 3 *The Clouds of War*
Book 4 *Redemption*
Book 5 *Betrayal*

With Edna Quammie

The Big House—Toronto General Hospital
Rainbow through the Rain
The *Qian Choi* Series
Prions from Wuhan
Die or Make Die
Rogue Pharma

Printed in Great Britain
by Amazon

26595367R00118